THERAPEUTIC CONSIDERATIONS for the ELDERLY

CLINICS IN PHYSICAL THERAPY
VOLUME 14

Forthcoming Volumes in the Series

THERAPEUTIC CONSIDERATIONS for the ELDERLY

Edited by

Osa Littrup Jackson, Ph.D.

Director and Associate Professor
  of Physical Therapy
Chairman, Department of Kinesiological Science
School of Health Sciences
Oakland University
Rochester, Michigan
Adjunct Assistant Professor
Physical Therapy Program
School of Health Related Professions
University of Pittsburgh
Pittsburgh, Pennsylvania

CHURCHILL LIVINGSTONE

NEW YORK, EDINBURGH, LONDON, MELBOURNE

1987

Library of Congress Cataloging-in-Publication Data

Therapeutic considerations for the elderly.

  (Clinics in physical therapy ; v. 14)
  Includes bibliographies and index.
  1. Physical therapy for the aged. I. Jackson, Osa.
II. Series. [DNLM: 1. Physical Therapy—in old age.
2. Rehabilitation—in old age. W1 CL831CN v.14 /
WB 460 T398]
RC953.8.P58T46   1987   615.8′2   87-9350
ISBN 0-443-08389-4

© **Churchill Livingstone Inc. 1987**

Distributed in the United Kingdom by Churchill Livingstone,
Robert Stevenson House, 1-3 Baxter's Place, Leith Walk,
Edinburgh EH1 3AF, and by associated companies, branches,
and representatives throughout the world.

Acquisitions Editor: *Kim Loretucci*
Copy Editor: *Julia Muiño*
Production Designer: *Rosalie Marcus*
Production Supervisor: *Jocelyn Eckstein*

Printed in the United States of America

First published in 1987

Contributors

Isabelle Bohman, M.S., P.T.
Physical Therapy Consultant, Breckenridge, Colorado

Gordon Burton, Ph.D., O.T.R.
Assistant Professor of Occupational Therapy, Department of Occupational Therapy, San Jose State University, San Jose, California; Clinician and Consultant, Partners in Learning Clinic, Carmichael, California

Elizabeth Dickinson, Ph.D.
Professor, Learning Resources Center, Michigan State University, East Lansing, Michigan

Dana Gage, M.D.
Attending Physician, Bellevue Emergency Services; Medical Director, Manhattan Veterans Administration Hospital, Hospital Based Home Care; Medical Director, Bellevue Hospital/Human Resources Administration Men's Shelter Clinic, New York, New York

Susan C. Hallenborg, M.Ed., P.T.
Clinical Instructor, Department of Rehabilitation Medicine, Tufts University School of Medicine, Boston, Massachusetts; Private Practitioner, Equipment Prescription Services, Billerica, Massachusetts

Osa Littrup Jackson, Ph.D.
Director, Associate Professor of Physical Therapy, and Chairman, Department of Kinesiological Science, School of Health Sciences, Oakland University, Rochester, Michigan; Adjunct Assistant Professor, Physical Therapy Program, School of Health Related Professions, University of Pittsburgh, Pittsburgh, Pennsylvania

Georgiana W. Johnson, M.A., R.P.T., C.C.C.
Private Practitioner, Boulder, Colorado

Lena Karlqvist, R.P.T.
Ergonomist and Consultant, Stockholm, Sweden

Tim Kauffman, M.S., P.T.
Private Practitioner, Byers, Kauffman, and Basciano Physical Therapy Rehabilitation, Lancaster, Pennsylvania

Margaret J. Leong, M.A., P.T.
Private Practitioner, Ossining, New York

Jacquelin Perry, M.D.
Professor of Orthopedic Surgery and Physical Therapy, University of Southern California School of Medicine, Los Angeles, California; Chief, Pathokinesiology Service, Rancho Los Amigos Hospital, Downey, California

Walter F. Pizzi, M.D.
Associate Professor of Clinical Surgery, Cornell University Medical Center; Chairman, Board of Directors, Regional Emergency Medical Services Council of New York City; Chairman, Department of Surgery, Catholic Medical Center of Brooklyn and Queens, New York, New York

Ruth B. Purtilo, Ph.D.
Professor and Chairperson, Department of Medical Jurisprudence and Humanities, University of Nebraska Medical Center, Omaha, Nebraska

Carola H. Speads
Instructor, Elsa Gindler Method of Physical Re-education, New York, New York

Jane St. Clair
Assistant Professor Adjunct, Health and Physical Education, Hunter College of the City University of New York; Executive Director, The Regional Emergency Medical Services Council of New York City, New York, New York

Darcy Umphred, Ph.D.
Clinician, Consultant, and Lecturer, Partners in Learning Clinic, Carmichael, California

Preface

This book describes the special skills needed to become a clinical specialist in geriatric physical therapy. The content is based on that in *Physical Therapy of the Geriatric Patient*, an earlier text in the <u>Clinics in Physical Therapy</u> series that summarizes the basic knowledge of gerontology and provides a rationale for adapting clinical interventions to meet the special needs of the geriatric patient. This volume introduces the clinical issues and describes in detail the unique modifications essential to adapting clinical intervention to the elderly. The premise is that geriatric rehabilitation and physical therapy will help each individual patient reach his full potential.

Central to the theme of this book are the belief in positive attitude and the willingness to continue learning. The "Foundation Concepts" purport that a person's age is not determined by his chronologic age. For instance, the chronologic age of a person does not regulate whether new skills—movement skills, interpersonal skills, self-awareness, and conceptual thinking—can be learned. The patient's real age is more directly related to how well he has adapted to life's challenges. The patient comes to physical therapy with medical, social, emotional, and/or cognitive disturbances and their secondary complications. Each patient needs to become aware of the personal, social, and environmental resources available to him for the ongoing improvement of adaptation to the demands of life. This is a lifelong process.

The second major concept presented here is that motivation is based on a sense of personal control. The therapeutic interaction must reinforce the patient's belief in his own ability to control the things in his life that make him happy and healthy. An important part of each treatment is to help strengthen the patient's internal locus of control (his sense of personal power).

The first three chapters introduce the Foundation Concepts, which provide the framework for clinical intervention for the elderly. In Chapter 1, a conceptual model is proposed for the process of geriatric rehabilitation. The model describes the emotional and physical responses that are the goals of therapeutic intervention and the measures to be taken to ensure the patient's successful progress. Each step in building the patient-therapist interaction is delineated. The model was designed as a checklist for geriatric rehabilitation to avoid unnecessary "backsliding," or loss of newly mastered skills. An important aspect of the model is the interface between physical therapy and restorative nursing which is the core component of a geriatric rehabilitation program.

Over time nearly every elderly person develops secondary complications (splinting, breath-holding on exertion, excessive muscular tension/rigidity, etc.), which, in most cases, can be appropriately managed by neurologic rehabilitation techniques.

The positive consequences that result when the therapist becomes aware of his patient's preferred style of learning and communicating are discussed in Chapter 2. While lack of motivation is often designated as the rationale for the termination of physical therapy and rehabilitation of an elderly patient, this chapter allows us another outcome. Neurolinguistic programming (NLP) is a clinical tool that formally recognizes that therapist and patient each have a preferred style for learning and communicating. An elderly patient comes to physical therapy with very low emotional and physical resources for adapting to the new environment, and it is unrealistic to expect him to adapt to the therapist's learning and communication style. Therefore, it is the physical therapist who must adapt. The first step in evaluation is to identify the patient's preferred learning and communication style. All interaction can then proceed on the patient's terms. The psychological support derived from this adjustment is likely to produce a more relaxed patient who can call on a store of emotional resources to carry out the physical therapy program. With the practice of NLP, the likelihood of creating a motivated and self-directed patient who reaches higher functional outcomes increases.

Chapter 3 presents a brief summary of the primary factors to be considered for effective use of neurologic rehabilitation techniques. The chapter also describes in detail the modifications necessary to allow the elderly patient to participate effectively in a program of neurologic rehabilitation.

Chapters 4 through 10 present Special Considerations, seven topics that were identified by practicing clinicians as the most important to address in an initial text on treatment modifications for the elderly. Chapter 4 presents the major modifications needed to facilitate ease and volume in ventilation and breathing in the elderly person. The premise is that enhancing breathing is possible in almost any individual despite the actual pathology or limitations of the physical structures. Facilitation of breathing is an important but separate component of neurologic rehabilitation. A rationale is presented for the use of these techniques as an initial warm-up to physical therapy. The belief is that as breathing and ventilation normalize, spontaneous improvements in movement and self-confidence occur. It is imperative that the reader understands that the brief description of the techniques is intended only as an introduction to breathing facilitation. To develop clinical mastery of the techniques, it is necessary to participate in laboratory course work.

Chapter 5 gives a general guideline for the safe use of heat and cold in physical therapy treatment of the elderly patient. A person's ability to monitor for overexposure to heat and cold is diminished with advanced age. A protocol that stipulates intensive monitoring of patient response is needed in using modalities that rely on the elderly patient's sensation of pain as an early indicator of overexposure. An interesting research study comparing temperature perceptions among young and old is included in the discussion.

Chapter 6 provides an overview of wheelchair adaptations commonly used for the severely disabled elderly. The topic was included at the request of clinicians who work with wheelchair-dependent elderly patients. A systematic review of the modifiable characteristics of a wheelchair is presented, and the interrelationships and complexities of wheelchair adaptations are highlighted. The importance of addressing the needs of each individual patient is stressed.

Chapter 7 presents the most common changes noted in the gait of elderly patients. An important item to note is that age alone contributes very little to alterations in gait, with no major functional disturbances resulting. The discussion focuses on the most common pathologies found in the gait of the elderly and implications for physical therapy intervention.

Chapter 8 includes an overview of the necessary modifications in administering cardiopulmonary resuscitation (CPR) to the elderly. The basic protocol for CPR was updated in June 1986, and the information in this chapter is based on those changes. Since about three-quarters of all heart attacks occur in the home, emergency procedures for CPR are an important consideration in the rehabilitation of the elderly. This patient population has shown consistently better functional results in a rehabilitation program that acknowledges the value of the patient remaining in his home for as long as possible. The chapter is intended as a quick reference for emergency procedures for the physical therapist working in the home care environment and highlights the importance of family education for the high-risk elderly cardiac patient.

Chapter 9 summarizes the most common functional losses seen in the long-term institutionalized elderly and sets down practical recommendations for the design of a living environment that maximizes independence in the elderly. The chapter is based on the findings of a study commissioned by the Swedish government, the goals of which were to examine functional losses present in patients residing in the skilled nursing home setting. With a tabulation of the most common functional losses, the researchers developed modifications of environmental organization and dimensions to achieve improved patient independence. This chapter emphasizes the desirability of compatible specialty equipment (e.g., bed and wheelchair).

A thoughtful discussion about the ethical considerations in geriatric rehabilitation is presented in Chapter 10, including those factors in the health care delivery system likely to make the elderly more vulnerable to emotional and/or physical neglect. A variety of supportive strategies that need to be considered in an effort to protect the elderly patient's rights are presented.

Two discussions of therapeutic modifications for physical therapy of the elderly patient are presented in Chapters 11 and 12. Chapter 11 was developed from an interview with Berta Bobath conducted in August 1985 in London. The conversation focused on the most important considerations and adaptations for the clinical management of the elderly patient. The transcripts of the interview were then presented to Isabelle Bohman, who refined the material as presented here. The thrust of the chapter re-emphasizes the fact that work with the elderly is worthwhile, and that the functional improvements resulting from physical therapy intervention can be significant.

In Chapter 12, a conceptual model for movement re-education in the well elderly (as well as younger persons) is presented. The program is a structured experience that develops each component of a movement and then facilitates the integration of the component's movements into functional activity. The concept of the Progressive Exercise Program (PEP) is based on life-long learning. The program lends itself equally well to movement re-education/refinement for senior athletes as well as for mildly disabled younger athletes. It is important to note that when used in the elderly patient, this program, as well as NDT, requires the individualizing of the therapy's demands to the needs of each patient. Thus, the effective clinical implementation of PEP and NDT mandates advanced training on the part of the physical therapist.

During my efforts to publish this work, numerous people were helpful and encouraging. There were many workshop participants who lobbied for the development of this text, and as the conceptual framework for the book developed, a number of clinicians helped me sharpen the focus of the book. I thank them for their support. My friend, Ruth Beckman Murray, has been a sounding board on the nursing/physical therapy interrelationship, and I gratefully acknowledge her help. An exciting aspect of developing this book was the chance to work with two senior clinicians, Berta Bobath and Carola Speads. These two women embody my personal goal of growing older and continuing to learn as well as to teach. I thank them for their inspiration. Special thanks go to the contributors for their thoughtful contributions. As the editor, I feel that I have learned a great deal from them and this experience. Lastly, I would like to thank David C. Gardner and Grace Joely Beatty for their thought-provoking work that has helped me to refine my personal feelings about growing older.

An acknowledgment goes to the innovators of a new conceptual model for geriatric rehabilitation in Hudiksval, Sweden. Their dream is partially my own: It *is* possible to create a health care delivery system where the value of home-based care would be acknowledged and highlighted. There are two important reasons for this goal: (1) recruiting and maintaining staff in nursing homes appears to be a worldwide problem and (2) the majority of elderly patients appear to function better with a rehabilitation program that acknowledges the desire to continue to live at home. The preliminary data have been collected and the Hudiksval project is accomplishing the desired goal: It is possible without increasing costs noticeably to change the process of health care delivery so that the patient can avoid unnecessary institutionalization and enjoy ongoing independence in their familiar home environment. Geriatric rehabilitation and effective health care delivery models are in their infancy but the refinements toward ideal care are an important goal.

The creation of this book represents my growing awareness of the interrelationship between health, wellness, and geriatric rehabilitation (physical, emotional, cognitive, social, and environmental). Those who facilitated my personal growth are Nils Klykken, my son, Marius, my mother and father, Raquel Olsen, Ella Ursin Steen, Grethe Øverli, Brit Hammel Malt, Guri Østby Damsløra, and Tove Sandvik. Through their caring, each of them helped me to grow and expand as a motivated, excited, and loving human being.

Osa (Aase) Littrup Jackson, Ph.D.

Contents

1 | Basic Principles in Rehabilitation: A Conceptual Model

Osa Littrup Jackson

> If we do not know what we are actually enacting then we cannot possibly do what we want.
>
> —Moshe Feldenkrais (1904–1984)

In rehabilitation of the geriatric patient, health professionals interact with people, real people like your mother or your grandmother. A person is referred to rehabilitation training due to some difficulty in their ability to carry out their desired daily activities. For many reasons, geriatric rehabilitation requires a collaborative interaction between the patient/meaningful others and a group of health professionals who are *interdependent* on each other (if the patient's best interests are to be served). With these concepts as the foundation, the specific interaction between the physical therapist/occupational therapist (PT/OT) and the patient/meaningful others* will be explored through the presentation of a conceptual model (see Fig. 1-1). The content of this chapter represents the

---

* Patient/meaningful others is presented as an inseparable unit since the goal of rehabilitation is to work toward normalization of the patient's lifestyle. The patient's network for emotional support must be actively involved in the total rehabilitation program. The outcome of focusing on the patient and his or her meaningful others as a unit is prevention of unnecessary secondary complications such as a family that feels unprepared or anxious about the patient returning to the home setting or a patient who feels isolated and excluded from the emotional support that is important to a sense of well-being).

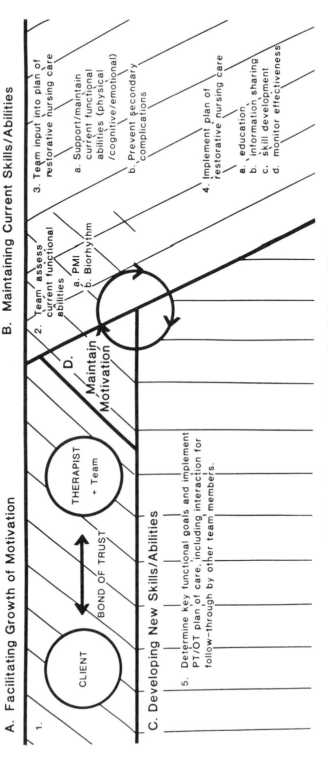

Fig. 1-1. The conceptual model of geriatric rehabilitation.

collaborative input of more than 400 health professionals (PT, OT, registered nurse) who attended my workshops in 1985 during summer/fall. To begin the discussion, each participant was asked to write a short description of the general goals of intervention with the elderly patient and any important comments in regard to the best way to achieve the desired outcome(s). The goal of this discussion was to develop a clear statement of intention/purpose in geriatric rehabilitation and in this way create a tool for checking that we stay on the therapeutic "track." A clear statement of intention can be thought of as a frame around a picture, since it delineates what variables clearly belong in the picture. The goal was to define the components and the natural limits of the therapeutic interaction.* It is important to note that the variables to be discussed will be presented in their natural order to show that there is a *sequential* order in the evolution of human movement and human potential.

The effectiveness of geriatric rehabilitation depends on the initial facilitation of motivation. Facilitation of the desire to participate (A in Fig. 1-1) and to try to help oneself is the cornerstone on which the entire treatment program is built. At the same time, from day 1, the effort to maintain current skills and abilities is initiated to the degree that the patient's motivational state allows. If it is feasible for at least one member of the team to develop a bond of trust with the client (that team member is then the primary liaison to the client), the primary focus of activity proceeds to an ongoing interaction of: efforts to maintain current skills/abilities (B in Fig. 1-1); efforts to develop new skills/abilities (C in Fig. 1-1); and efforts to maintain motivation (D in Fig. 1-1).

Ongoing monitoring is necessary in this circle of activities to assure that development of new skills is achieved concurrently with active support for the current skills of the patient. (For example, if a patient is learning ambulation skills, but in the evening has not reached the commode as quickly as needed and has bladder accidents constantly, the patient's motivation to participate in rehabilitation and in *all of life* will be seriously compromised.) Rehabilitation of the elderly is possible in many cases, but requires attention to the details of patient care.

THE ELDERLY PATIENT

The elderly patient has special needs, and it is for this reason that a new model for therapeutic interaction must be developed. With a young or middle-aged patient, it is usually safe to presume that the person has some ability to adapt to demands and to the new environment (except the patient in intensive care, recovery room, emergency room, or the patient with acute psychiatric problems). In large part PT/OT entry level training has focused on therapeutic

---

* Some types of interaction and nurturing from meaningful others can never be substituted for or replaced by therapeutic interaction. Therefore, supporting the desired role of the meaningful others is an important part of rehabilitation.

interaction with patients who were younger (under 65 years of age) and who had the presumed ability to adapt to some degree to the routine of the hospital or the clinical environment. The disease and/or conditions to be treated in the past usually involved only one isolated area of the body or a simple and clearly understood disease mechanism (ie, infection). Treatment strategies were developed along logical lines of thinking and led to predictable results. It was also presumed that the patient was at least minimally motivated.

The elderly patient is special since the life experiences that occur from age 60 to 100 years are uniquely different from those of other times of life. The later years are in large part characterized by major losses or changes in roles, income, self-image, and abilities.[2] The age-related changes often occur in clusters, and the person's abilities to adapt and to solve problems are therefore taxed to their limit. For example, it is not unusual for an elderly patient of 82 to have attended eight funerals, within the last year, of people who were of personal significance. Persons involved in a mourning process have a limited ability to adapt to new situations and new demands.[3] Elderly patients who come to rehabilitation are also in a major identity crisis or in mourning over the loss or distortion of physical, emotional, and cognitive abilities that has precipitated the need for the referral to rehabilitation. For all these reasons, initially, the elderly disabled person who is referred to PT/OT can be presumed to have very limited adaptive abilities and a questionable degree of motivation or desire to participate. The same geriatric patient will also usually have from three to 10 medical problems which must all be managed (the patient should follow the regimen that existed for the problems prior to the current crisis, if the problems are not directly involved with the crisis) while the acute medical problem(s) are being diagnosed and then treated.

LATERAL THINKING AND GERIATRIC REHABILITATION

In light of all the above-mentioned considerations, logical behavior, logical problem solving, and logical treatment programs are not always going to be the most effective strategies for working with the elderly patient. In geriatric rehabilitation, lateral thinking is a tool that can yield very positive clinical results. Lateral thinking is defined by the Oxford English Dictionary as:

> a way of thinking which seeks the solution of intractable problems through unorthodox methods or elements which would normally be ignored by logical thinking . . . lateral thinking leads to those simple ideas that are obvious only after they have been thought of.[4]

In traditional medical management of a knee problem of a young adult, it may be necessary to involve only the patient, the physician, and the PT. The treatment program involves logical vertical thinking: each step follows the next in an unbroken sequence, reasoning must be correct at every step, and only relevant information is considered. In management of a knee problem of an 82-year-old widow, it may be necessary to involve the patient, the physician, the OT, and perhaps 10 other individuals (daughter, neighbor, friend, PT, nurse, minister, social worker, etc.) to collect enough data that provides an overview of the patient's total situation. The father of lateral thinking, Edward de Bono, would describe this as the "PMI—a method for avoiding the intelligence trap . . . of jumping in and providing logical intervention."[5]

In the case of our 82-year-old patient, this would mean:

Step 1: *P* = *pluses*, tabulating the assets;

Step 2: *M* = *minuses*, tabulating the obvious minuses in the situation;

Step 3: *I* = *interesting*, listing those other pieces of information that are just interesting. The objective is to provide broadmindedness by delaying judgment. It is also helpful to use PMI as a way of delaying the addition of the personal emotional component by the members of the rehabilitation team.

In the case of the 82-year-old patient with a knee dysfunction, it may mean that the key to success in rehabilitation is to provide the following nursing plan of care:

To allow the patient to bathe herself even if it takes 1 hour daily (important to her);

To make sure she is dressed in her *habitual way** (ie, brassiere, girdle, hose, slip, and dress) in the morning with help as needed;

To put makeup on in her habitual way;

To have her hair done in her usual way;

To have her dressed in her *own* clothing;

To install a telephone by her bedside (with a lock so others cannot use it when she is out of the room). The rationale for providing the telephone is that all of the patient's meaningful others are unable to travel to visit her as often as she needs emotional support;

To have her wear her comfortable walking shoes when she is up;

To arrange a private room or else a roommate with similar bedtime and lifestyle (who is not confused or aggressive);

In addition to this, the patient's family would be asked to bring her dog to the facility daily and PT/OT would be scheduled twice daily.

The short-term goal is for the patient to be able to walk her dog as necessary and to take care of all the dog's needs. (The best possible solution is to have a kennel on the grounds of the facility with the patients, when able, in charge of all the care of pets–walking, feeding, etc.). The desired result is that in 2 weeks the patient is independently ambulating in a wheelchair for all needs,

---

* The habits of a lifetime in personal grooming and activities of daily living that are familiar and help to build and maintain self-confidence and high self-esteem.

which leads to an increase in motivation and self-esteem and, in 3 more weeks, is independently walking, with a walker, with her dog.

Lateral thinking often involves using a solution that is only obvious in retrospect (the strong motivation to care for a pet). In light of the limited number of pluses for many elderly patients and the large number of minuses, the variables that often point to the "therapeutic key" are the items that are listed as "interesting personal data." Thus, if a patient refuses all rehabilitation efforts but still goes to chapel or the beauty shop, the therapist should regard these aspects as important and interesting data that point to the "therapeutic key." Rehabilitation after severe illness or injury is possible for many elderly patients, but the way in which it is carried out must be customized to the unique resources and assets of each individual.

THE CONCEPTUAL MODEL

Bond of Trust (Fig. 1-2)

Many things are not obvious. Most psychotherapies use speech to get to unconscious, forgotten, early experiences. Yet feelings go on in ourselves long before speech is learned. Some pay attention not to what is said, but to how it is said. Doing this enables one to find the *intentions* behind the structure of the phrasing, so that one can get to the feelings that dictated the particular way of phrasing. In short, how one says what one does is at least as important as what one does.

—Moshe Feldenkrais

When the therapist and the patient meet, a bond of trust must develop between them before the two can express their full potential in interaction. The elusive obvious is that if attention is paid to the details of creating the bond of trust, the intention of rehabilitation can be carried out in the most effective way. As described by one of the earliest supporters of rehabilitation, it is a process that has very clear desired outcomes:

Generally speaking, all parts of the body which have a function, if used in moderation, and exercised in labors to which each is accustomed, becomes thereby healthy and well developed, and age slowly; but if unused and left idle, they become liable to disease, defective in growth, and age quickly. This is especially the case with joints and ligaments, if one does not use them. In those who are neglected and never use the leg to walk with, but keep it up in the air, the bones are more atrophied than in those who do use it; and the tissues are much more atrophied than in those who use the leg.

—Socrates

The goal of therapeutic interaction is to bring patients to their highest level

Facilitating Growth of Motivation

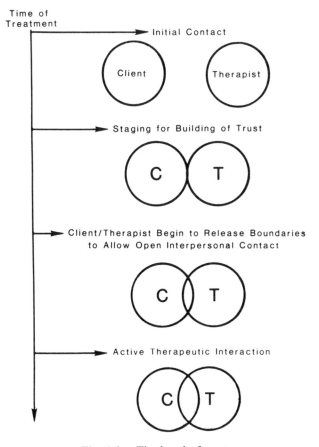

Fig. 1-2. The bond of trust.

of functional abilities while preventing unnecessary secondary complications. The major question that has never been clearly addressed is identification of the person who should decide what the most important functional abilities are for a particular patient. Every human being defines his or her identity based on certain abilities, and the individuality of the definition is what makes that person who he or she is. For one client, a pivotal ability for maintaining self-esteem, identity, and sense of personal value is the ability to wash dishes (and thereby contribute to the smooth operation of a household), whereas, for another person the ability to walk may be the core of identity. The feelings related to self-worth and self-esteem exist whether the patient can express them in speech or not. For this reason, the first step in clarifying the *intention* of rehabilitation is to state: *patients are the ones who must provide the decisive input about what is most important to their ability to maintain their sense of self-worth and identity.* In other words, the therapist must interact in such a way that the intention of rehabilitation is expressed by every action of the therapist and other members of the rehabilitation team. The clear message that the patient needs to hear is:

1. You the patient are accepted as you are.
2. Your input is essential to the best outcome for your rehabilitation.
3. Your feeling of being in control of your life is important.
4. You, the patient, have certain basic feelings about what is most important to you, and the rehabilitation team is open to interacting with you on your terms.

If therapeutic interaction is built on these ideas, the necessary bond of trust between the patient and the therapist (rehabilitation team) is given an ideal foundation from which to grow.

In light of these basic premises, developing a treatment program for the geriatric patient involves a new emphasis. The decisive data for determining the best plan of care/therapy for a patient begin with the category of information that de Bono calls interesting, or a list of all the information that at the moment is no more than interesting because it only helps to describe the individuality of the person who is the patient. This can also be described as initiating the stage of building the bond of trust (see Fig. 1-2).

Every effort, every contact, with the patient in geriatric rehabilitiation must be based on the intention of respecting the personal dignity and self-worth of the patient. The elderly patient is special; thus, the therapist initially must adapt to meet the individual needs of each patient, since this patient population often has very limited adaptive skills/resources when entering the rehabilitation program. (Once the bond of trust is developed, most elderly patients appear to have good potential for positive rehabilitation outcomes.) The bond of trust between the therapist and the patient grows from the patient's feeling of: (1) acceptance of his or her individuality, including loss of vision or hearing, a need for altered teaching styles, etc., and, (2) the respect for his or her continued (human) need to maintain personal dignity and self-worth (especially related to habits of personal grooming, dress, hair style, makeup, biorhythm-bedtimes, religion, biases, etc.).

Practical Issues in Building the Bond of Trust

If the bond of trust develops, it is as though the client/therapist begin to release the personal boundaries, and in this way allow deeper interpersonal sharing and ease. Once a bond of trust is established as a part of the initial PMI and assessment of functional abilities, it is an ongoing task to nurture and build this foundation for human interaction.

The bond of trust between the patient and the therapist is influenced by two major categories of activities: (1) the total environment in which the care is given (see Chapter 9) and, (2) the special adaptations that the therapist can make that will help the patient to feel accepted and more secure. The practicality of achieving real geriatric rehabilitation (physical therapy treatment included) begins with focusing on the details of *how* the most mundane tasks are performed. The elusive obvious is that real geriatric rehabilitation can only occur in an environment where the basic activities of daily living (ADL) (bathing; grooming; selecting clothes; putting on clothes or participating in combing hair, dressing, putting on jewelry, or applying makeup; serving food; eating; attending to toilet functions and needs, etc.) are done in a way that supports the patient's individuality, personal dignity, and sense of safety and comfort.

Many of the aspects of the therapeutical milieu are maintained by the nursing staff of the institution, but the PT and OT may act in a consulting role (eg, by obtaining furniture that is functional for the aged patient or by giving input about color or other esthetic features).

The therapeutic goal is therefore to work toward (the work is an ongoing process which can always be made better) establishing normal expectations about daily activities. As this might relate to eating lunch, it would mean a normalized environment (a place where the usual roles and personal options are possible), for example:

1. The ability to choose for oneself at the moment—the patient can choose one scoop or two of potatoes or have a second helping.
2. A safe environment with no fear of others intruding on the place of eating (confused or disoriented patients are provided with special eating assistance or time or place of eating that does not disrupt the mealtime for other alert patients).
3. The ability to sit with one's choice of people with the option of family or friends being able to participate or to sit alone as one wishes.
4. Being given a reasonable amount of time and physical help (as needed) to carry out the chosen activity.
5. Having a physical environment that provides the needed space (accessibility between tables, for getting in and out with a wheelchair, cane(s), walker).
6. Appropriate lighting (without glare).
7. Visually attractive surroundings that are comfortable for the target population—patients. In addition, the furniture is as functional as possible (ie, dining room chairs provide armrests to assist the patient in standing, and the height of the chair seat is suited to the height of the average patient (in many long-term care facilities the height would be 5 feet or less). Persons who are 5ft 5in to 6ft 5in are provided with chairs suitable to their individual height.
8. Respect for ethnic values in food, dress, music, etc.

These concepts, fostered by nursing, can then be reinforced by the PT and OT working closely with the nursing staff and supported in their contact with the administrators of the institution. Often, the requests made by the nursing staff (eg, for certain kinds of furniture or use of certain colors, art work, lighting effects, etc.) need the reinforcement of other members of the therapeutic team to highlight the physiological rationale for the requests. The people most involved with care of the patient should have input in decisions that affect patients and their care. This is a factor to be dealt with not only in the rehabilitation setting but also in any institutional setting.

To facilitate a good night's rest, the basics of the policy and procedure manual would address such questions as the need for:

1. A quiet and undisturbed environment, unless it is an absolute medical emergency, (ie, no paging over loudspeaker at night, staff shoe soles made of material to promote quiet walking, staff discussions carried out away from patient's sleeping area etc.)

2. An absolute sense of personal safety and ease: (a) not having to worry about a confused patient coming in and claiming that the bed is his or hers; and (b) being allowed to lock the door at night and having an aide who will enter in response to a call—that is, be required to knock and, unless it is an emergency, wait for permission to enter,

3. A respect for pillow, mattress, blankets, and pajama habits (since a lifetime of personal experiences has determined what is individually best.)

4. Lighting that is workable, taking into consideration the patient's current functional abilities (see Chapter 9, ie, grip strength), and that is adequate to allow safety for independent toileting (if functionally possible).

5. Temperature that is acceptable to the habits of the patient to allow for quality sleep (ease of temperature regulation, access to fresh air, minimum of draft).

6. Access to refreshments (coffee, tea, etc.) and habitual night activities—patient lounge open, etc.).

7. Ease of access to a safe, pleasant outdoor area as would be habitual for patient (ie, evening stroll in garden—all year in warm climate or only in summer in colder regions).

Again, the nursing staff is responsible for maintaining this milieu, but the PT/OT will want to receive assurance from the nursing staff that the geriatric rehabilitation patient has the advantage of the environment described.

The bond of trust grows from the patients' feelings that their needs and wishes are viewed as important and taken seriously. Physiologically, the same policies and procedure items that have been mentioned will also decrease unnecessary anxiety and transplantation shock. The desired outcome is achieved when the patient is getting restful and sound sleep, a pivotal factor in the patient's ability to perform effectively in all rehabilitation activities. A patient experiencing sleep difficulty who previously did not have any problems in sleeping may simply be manifesting a symptom that is related to stress/anxiety.[7]

Physical or occupational therapists who desire to work with the elderly must be prepared to work as a part of a total geriatric rehabilitation team that has three major tasks: (1) to maintain and support the patient's self-worth and positive self-esteem; (2) to develop and maintain a sense of personal safety for the patient, including the bond of trust with members of the team; and (3) use

(A) and (B) (see Figure 1) as precursors to the actual PT/OT intervention that is designed to improve and maximize the patient's functional abilities.

Home Based Care: Ideal Environment for Building the Bond of Trust

The frail elderly patient will, in most cases, tend to gain emotional strength and self-confidence from living in his or her habitual dwelling (own home), in which the patient will have a "built-in" sense of mastery and control over an environment by nature of having lived there for a long time with familiar possessions.

It is very difficult to control all the variables in the institutional environment of care to assure the patient a sense of control and mastery. For most elderly patients, it is usually easier for the PT/OT to exert maximal control over the environmental variables (so that they support the intent of rehabilitation) in the patient's own home. There are exceptions related to problems between patient and caregiver, poor safety in the home, etc. It is well known that, given a choice, most patients prefer to live in their own homes and not in an institution. Today, the United States appropriates 7 to 8 percent of the total health care budget to provide services in a home-care setting. Is this enough to support the intent to provide effective home-based geriatric rehabilitation for high-risk and frail elderly? Who is to be the advocate for home-based geriatric rehabilitation? These questions are raised as a springboard for discussion, and it is obvious that a resolution that will support the desires of the elderly and the disabled will take time to develop.

Research performed at TRIAGE and other pilot programs indicates that home-based geriatric rehabilitation is no more expensive than institutional-based care; in some cases, it is cheaper.[8] A major difference noted in the home-based geriatric rehabilitation programs was that the patient/meaningful others expressed a greater sense of ease and more satisfaction with the program of care. On the other hand, the elderly patient who is perceived in the institution as irreversibly handicapped will, through a home care rehabilitation program, recover more physiological function than was ever thought possible. There are, however, exceptions to this. The frail aged person may have no remaining meaningful others either living nearby or able to live with them or to assist them with some of the tasks of daily living. Sometimes the frail aged cannot be rehabilitated beyond a certain point physically, cognitively, or emotionally and, in their state of dependency, may feel more secure in the institution, which has structure yet acknowledges individuality and unique needs. Some elderly people choose to go to a structured living arrangement prior to the time that frailty occurs.

Communication and Fostering Trust

Therapists can adapt their behavior and verbal communication to that of the client, in this case the elderly client. There are many ways to develop the bond of trust so necessary for a therapeutic environment. One of the most obvious ways, but, paradoxically, one that is seldom used, is to pay attention to the client's primary learning style. Usually, however, the therapist is unaware not only of the client's learning style but of her or his own; what results is a breakdown in communication and, therefore, trust. As therapists, we blame this breakdown on the clients "just being old" or even on "senility" when, in truth, it has to do with our communication skills. Neurolinguistic Programming (NLP) offers the therapist a set of tools to recognize his or her primary learning or communication style and that of the client's and attempts to match the two (see Chapter 2).

According to NLP, people have three common learning styles: visual, auditory, and kinesthetic. Some individuals have the ability to learn easily in any of the three learning styles, but most of us tend to have one favored style; if information is not communicated in that style, we can initially experience confusion instead of understanding. The learning style is reflected in our choice of words, eye movements, and movement patterns. If an elderly client is primarily a visual learner and the therapist is an auditory learner, they can be like two ships passing in the night. Rapport and trust can be slow to develop; suddenly, the patient may catch on to how the therapist talks or perhaps, particularly in the case of an elderly patient who is experiencing grief or mourning, understanding may never occur. NLP provides the therapists with a systematic and precise approach to gaining the necessary clinical skills for immediately recognizing and adapting their learning mode to those of their clients, by teaching therapists to (a) determine their own and the patient's favored/habitual learning style, and (b) adapt their style of communication and teaching to the way that is easiest and most familiar for the patient, thereby building the bond of trust.

The bond of trust that results from good communication is often the "therapeutic key" that unlocks the client's ability to participate in his or her own health care program. The client who feels a bond of trust with the therapist chooses to participate and to contribute energy and effort to accomplishing the mutually agreed-on goals and valued functional activities and habits closely linked to self-worth. The elderly client with a sense of self-worth is most likely to reach their potential when the predominant learning style of a patient is determined through assessment and it is imperative that this knowledge be shared with the rest of the team. Furthermore, an education program should then be set up so that all team members use the same approach consistently in responding to the patient's predominant learning style. It is presumed that work of this kind is built on first orienting staff to assessing their own learning styles and what this means to the process of communication.

III. Maintaining Current Functional Skills/Abilities (Figure 1-B)

The maintenance of current functional skills/abilities hinges on three major activities: (1) team assessment of current functional skills (including physical/occupational therapy); (2) team input into the restorative nursing plan of care;

(including physical/occupational therapy); and (3) implementation of a restorative nursing plan of care and monitoring of the effectiveness of these efforts.

The rationale is that if rehabilitation efforts do nothing else, they must support the basic intent of any intervention—to do no harm.

Assessment

A client's assessment provides a baseline—a clear description of the patient's emotional, physical, and cognitive skills and abilities (see B2 in Fig. 1-1). A subordinate goal of rehabilitation (assigned most often as a restorative nursing responsibility) is to maintain/support the current functional skills of the client as documented by the team assessment.

Rehabilitation is built on the premise that active support exists to maintain current skills as the new and desired skills evolve through specific treatments by PT/OT, speech, psychological intervention, etc. The assessment data is immediately organized so that: (1) the client's abilities are itemized, and successes are highlighted; (2) current skills and abilities are actively supported through every detail of staff–patient interaction; and (3) current skills and abilities are used as the platform from which to build the bond of trust needed for effective rehabilitation results.

For the elderly, because of their commonly high levels of stress prior to entering the rehabilitation program, assessment is always made simultaneously with the first step of treatment, nurturing/facilitating motivation (the desire to do for oneself—to take charge). Assessment in physical and occupational therapy is unique among many other disciplines because the assessment not only measures or quantifies what currently exists but measures and assesses the *neurological plasticity or potential* for improvements in functional abilities. For example, for the physical therapist, assessment of ability in performing ADL (ie, transferring from wheelchair to bed) may include assessment of: (1) the patient's ease of breathing, rhythm, rate of breathing while sitting; (2) the patient's response to facilitation to promote normalization/maximization of ease of breathing; (3) the patient's posture in the sitting position; (4) the patient's response to facilitation to promote normalization of posture; (5) the patient's active use of limbs; (6) the patient's response to *facilitation** to normalize/maximize controlled use of limbs; (7) the patient's motor planning to execute actual transfer from wheelchair to bed; (8) the patient's active transfer from wheelchair to bed; (9) the suitability of equipment involved—bed, wheelchair, sliding board, bed linen, etc. The PT/OT assessment can therefore yield data that can be categorized using PMI:

---

* The term facilitation is used in a broad sense to describe any therapeutic stimulus designed to create an improved performance in functional ability.

P—Pluses

Pluses are those activities that respond or appear to show improvement with facilitation/therapeutic intervention. The pluses indicate that treatment focused on this movement/skill are likely to lead to improved levels of performance.

M—Minuses

Minuses are those structural losses/movement distortions that initially appear unresponsive during assessment of ability (with or without facilitation). One therapist can often reveal patients' abilities that were not previously obvious to another therapist. Our energy level/individuality/personality learning-teaching style as a therapist are as important in performing therapy as our professional skills.

I—Interesting

All data that cannot clearly be categorized as a plus or minus, but are more relevant to describing the individuality of the client are termed interesting.

Biorhythm

To help maintain current skills and abilities, assessment of the elderly patient also must consider a person's biorhythm. An 82-year-old client has a lifetime of habits related to the time of day of performing activities and the sequencing of specific activities. It is not unusual to find some people who are morning people, who enjoy getting up at 5:00 a.m. and who have done so for 60 years. One goal of the rehabilitation team is to *utilize consciously each client's biorhythm* to support a positive and therapeutically desired outcome. An elderly client who is already under severe emotional and physical stress may find that requirements of adapting to a drastically different bedtime and rising time and an alteration of the sequencing of rest, mild, moderate, and maximal physical activity and emotional/cognitive stimulation can cause or contribute to acute dementia or transplantation shock. The symptoms are development of cognitive dysfunction over a short period of time; acute dementia is reversible if the overstimulation (demand for adaptive skills) is removed or altered and the client is allowed to return to a familiar, personally desirable environment with appropriate help for the transition.[10] In all cases, if the return to the familiar environment is to be a success, it must happen as soon as possible after the onset of symptoms.

The frail elderly represent a challenge to rehabilitation programs since the timing and sequencing of activities, if done in a pattern familiar to the patient, often leads to great improvements in functional abilities. The focus on bio-rhythms is most important when a patient is making the transition from a home environment to a hospital or nursing home (for temporary or permanent place-ment). A schedule of daily activity that is familiar to the total physiological makeup of the patient is likely to allow the patient to perform best in rehabi-litation. If the team wishes to change a client's daily activity and sleep rhythm, this should be done purposefully and at a pace that is physiologically and psy-chologically sound for the client (unnecessary complications, ie, acute dementia and stress symptoms such as urinary frequency, waking up in the middle of the night and unable to go to sleep again, etc. can be avoided).[11]

When possible, the patient should be allowed to go to sleep and to rise at a time in keeping with the lifetime schedule. Medications should be limited to those that are absolutely essential; those that calm the central nervous system (CNS), such as tranquilizers and sedatives, should be omitted for physiological and psychological reasons. Depressant medications given to a person who is at the low point of the biorhythm cycle, make the person even more sleepy, sedated, ataxic, and apparently unmotivated. Furthermore, the patient's ther-apy should be instituted when the biorhythm is at a high point rather than at low point so that maximal effect can be obtained from therapeutic efforts.

The ambulatory elderly person who must get up at night to urinate is aided by having adequate lighting to safely move from bed to restroom. Nursing staff should note the usual time of voiding of those patients who require assistance so that the patient will not struggle alone, possibly falling in the attempt.

PT/OT/Nursing Interaction

The professional nurse/nursing aide staffing pattern and level of aide training of nursing service is a pivotal variable in the entire discussion of maintenance of current skills/abilities for each patient. If professional nursing staff or nursing aides are too few in number or if aides have inadequate or inconsistent training, it is not possible to continue the efforts begun in PT/OT or to delegate the responsibility of maintaining current skills/abilities solely to the restorative nursing plan of care. A PT/OT who is considering employment at any medical facility must look at the staffing support that exists in nursing both in terms of actual manpower and the level of training. If nursing is not fully and consistently staffed, a large part of PT/OT activities will be focused primarily on supporting and supplementing the restorative nursing plan of care. If there is not adequate nursing aide staffing, PT/OT will focus primarily on maintaining and supporting current skills and abilities. Without adequate nursing manpower, the role of physical therapy may include:

1. Transfer of patients who need assistance onto the toilet. PT should be scheduled at the usual time of the patient's bowel movement if possible, to assure an adequate amount of help in transferring the patient comfortably and safely.

2. Timing the treatment for skill development so that it coincides with the needed restorative nursing function and so that there is no loss of motivation related to problems or fears about reaching the bathroom in time.

3. Teaching current nursing staff the easiest way to transfer such a patient; all PT training must thus be refocused to the most essential ADL skills for assuring personal dignity and a sense of control and safety (bathroom skills, transfer skills, eating skills, and basic wheelchair mobility skills).

4. Acting as consultant to be available whenever nursing staff experience problems with moving a patient in bed, transferring a patient or assisting a patient in bathroom functions. Emphasis is placed on being able to provide every patient, (your mother or grandmother) with a dignified and comfortable experience in getting in and out of bed and on and off the toilet. Maslow's theory of hierarchy of needs implies that if the client does not feel at ease with these two basic needs (bathroom functions and bed transfers) there is no chance for facilitating motivation to participate in a rehabilitation program or *in life*.

The bottom line is that without an adequate program (staffing level and training level) of restorative nursing, physical therapy has little time left to focus on the most fruitful part of the therapeutic interaction—building new and necessary skills for the patient, presuming that current skills (physical, emotional, and cognitive) are consciously maintained through the restorative nursing plan of care. If restorative nursing is not operational:

1. The patient's current skills and abilities are usually not adequately maintained.

2. Physical therapy treatment becomes focused on primarily restorative nursing tasks (maintaining bathroom function, dressing, and mobility for the patient).

3. There is usually inadequate practice time to reinforce skill development on the nursing unit; thus, the nurse or aide may do for the patient rather than allow the patient to *practice* (so essential to all mastery of new motor skills and building of self-confidence).

The team assessment is carried out simultaneously as the bond of trust develops between the patient and the team members. If the bond of trust is not developing within 2 to 3 days, a systematic effort to support the development of the bond of trust must be instituted. *Geriatric rehabilitation cannot occur if a bond of trust does not exist between the patient and at least one of the providers of care.* The assessment in most cases allows each team member to quantify the patient's current abilities and skills and at the same time lay the foundation for the bond of trust. The list of current skills and abilities gives the patient, family, and staff a list of skills they can draw on and utilize. For the patient, the ability to use available skills and abilities is a source of pride, supporting healthy self-esteem. For the family (meaningful others), the awareness of the things that the patient can do and the need to practice can give a starting point for defining how they can *best* help, that is, interact with the patient in a way that helps the patient build self-confidence. For the staff, the investment of time it takes to itemize the client's skills and abilities means that individualized restorative nursing care is possible. The staff that actively works at assessing and supporting the patient's current skills and abilities promote: (1) a patient who needs more supervision (teaching) and less of the actual doing for the patient; (2) a patient who is doing for himself or herself; a patient tends to be in better spirits. Restorative nursing philosophy is built on the premise that a patient needs time to practice skills in daily activities (not just in PT/OT) if they are to be mastered as a useful habit pattern and retained as a skill.

Team Input Into Restorative Nursing Plan of Care

Although the nursing staff is ultimately responsible for the nursing care plan, other team members may contribute ideas (see B3 in Fig. 1-1). The goals of allowing each member of the rehabilitation team (including the patient/meaningful others) to participate in refining and individualizing the restorative nursing plan of care are:

1. To be assured that all interaction with the patient respects and supports the individuality of the person;

2. To be assured that the patient's sense of self-determination and control are not compromised (more than is personally tolerable) to expedite a desired rehabilitation outcome;

3. To be sure that the family/meaningful others are tapped for those resources they are able to provide, and that they are included in the ongoing rehabilitation program (made to feel welcome and useful);

4. To insure that a complete description of current skills and abilities (physical, ADL, emotional, cognitive, etc.), from the perspective of the PT/OT, is made available to the nursing staff who will be interacting most with the patient.

5. To emphasize that a restorative nursing plan of care implies that the nursing staff function primarily in the teaching/assisting role. The more accurate the assessment and reassessment, the more the staff will be able to work on maintaining/using the patient's current skills and abilities, and having the patient do the necessary practice in ADL on the nursing unit following instructions given in physical and occupational therapy.

6. To insure the interplay of all data collected by each team member and provide a way to check the accuracy of the restorative and nursing care plan and areas of inconsistency that occur.

7. To delineate openly those ADL tasks that the patient currently can perform (these abilities are the key to the patient's self-image) or physiological status, and to delineate how the nursing staff will take responsibility for maintaining those skills. This approach allows room for nursing staff to indicate that on the day shift a staff member who is competent at helping to put on an above-

knee prosthesis is available, but that no one with this expertise is available in the afternoons. The task of helping the client perform bathroom functions while wearing a prosthesis and to remove it, will have to be taught as a PT/OT training function on the unit, with the participation of the patient and afternoon/evening personnel. The goal at all times is to work to create support so that the patient does not lose those skills and abilities he or she possesses while new skills are being developed. Abilities develop sequentially. If the patient is fearful, angry, or frustrated about bathroom activities, motivation for all other life activities is usually negatively affected.

8.   To allow input based on the assessment results in the sequencing of activities with the hope of being able to organize a physiologically comfortable transition in the patient's biorhythm when necessary. Reinforcing a person's habitual biorhythm by organizing rehabilitation care around it, thus allowing the patient to function maximally, is an obvious asset.

9.   To highlight the effective patient outcomes.

A clear delineation of the patient's current abilities and skills will provide the best foundation for a restorative nursing plan of care. Each member of the rehabilitation team has unique abilities which, combined with interpersonal skills, will permit observation and identification of different assets in the patient. The sharing of data by team members assures a therapeutically effective rehabilitation program.

Implementing the Restorative Nursing Plan of Care

Implementation of the restorative nursing plan of care for each patient organizes who does what, when, where, and how (see B4 in Fig. 1-1). In addition to the patient, three major groups are involved in a restorative nursing plan of care; they are the nursing staff, other staff as responsibilities are delegated (PT, OT, speech, social work, recreation, visits from clergymen, etc.), and family/ meaningful others. The goal of the restorative nursing plan of care is to maximize the patient's current abilities and to work systematically to maintain the patient's motivation to work toward new and needed skills. Implementation of the restorative nursing plan of care for a patient usually involves four distinct activities: (1) information sharing, (2) education, (3) skill development, and (4) monitoring of effectiveness.

To implement a nursing plan of care, *basic information sharing* is needed to develop the organizational framework. The first step involves notifying the necessary people of their roles, explaining the rationale, scheduling activities at the most effective time, deciding on the easiest way, and brainstorming to develop other options; all this is part of the scope of information sharing. Accountability is a key concept. For each item of information sharing, the chart should reflect who is taking responsibility, what the goal of the information sharing is, and when it will be completed; it should also reflect any special instructions or precautions. The goal at all times is to be able, as a rehabilitation team, to state the patient's current skills and abilities and then, in detail, itemize what the team has done, what the team is in the process of doing, and what the team hopes to do to support the client's ability to maintain his or her current level of skills (physical, psychological, social).

The second step in implementing the nursing plan of care is activation of any *formal education/training*. The goal of educational activities is to prepare the staff (nursing and other) as well as the family/meaningful others, to be capable of helping the patients feel safe and motivated to do as much as possible for themselves. For example, a formal program can train staff and the family/meaningful others of an elderly woman to recognize the warning signs of overexertion so that they will not overprotect the patient and do too much for her. Assume that a patient has recently recovered from bypass surgery and has been ill for more than a year. It is possible that the patient may become completely independent, but on admission to the nursing home she needs help to bathe her feet and back and slight help in dressing. The patient now performs these activities at a slow pace but must take rest breaks every 5 to 6 minutes and just stop. The family prefers that the patient not overexert and the staff prefer to get bathing and dressing done in a faster time. What is best for the patient? The patient is extremely pleased with her new-found endurance which, she notes, is improving. The patient needs to practice her ADL skills (slowly) to maintain current abilities and to gain new endurance. The fear and over-protection on the part of the family creates much frustration and distress for the patient. The education is the foundation on which staff and family can justify the behavior that ultimately will be best for the patient's rehabilitation outcome, letting the patient do as much as she feels is comfortable for her.

The third step involves *skill building* on the part of staff and family that will make the patient's activities as safe as possible. For a patient who is able to transfer from wheelchair to toilet or bed with verbal cueing and standby physical assistance, skill building will involve the nursing aides as well as family. The nurse or aide who can verbally cue in the proper sequence and can guard the patient will give the patient the valuable practice needed to maintain current skills. The family member who feels confident in verbal cueing and guarding will be more likely to invite the patient to go for an outing or home for a visit. Family members who have been involved in training can feel that they have something real to contribute that is a valuable support to their loved one. The patient will feel safer and more confident when all staff and family are able to provide consistent and appropriate help.

The last part of a restorative nursing plan of care involves the *ongoing process of monitoring for changes*. To monitor, the nursing staff must know the patient in order to recognize small changes and early warning signs. In the average health care facility, elderly patients will need primary nursing. The precision and effectiveness in monitoring and supporting the patient's current abilities is built, in large part, on the bond of trust or therapeutic relationship between the nursing staff and the patient. In geriatric rehabilitation, the better the bond of trust between the patient and the staff, the greater the chance of monitoring and supporting the patient's current abilities.

Developing New Skills/Abilities

On the foundation of the bond of trust between the patient and the rehabilitation team, the team assessment and the restorative nursing plan of care is developed and implemented. At this time, an active program is in place to prevent "backsliding" of functional skills and secondary complications (see C in Fig. 1-1). With these prerequisites established, a physical therapy treatment program will have the greatest chance of a successful outcome, unique to each patient and defined as those special skills and key functional goals that enhance the patient's quality of life in the most significant way. Developing new skills provides needed support for maintaining motivation and increasing adaptability (see D in Fig. 1-1). The PT treatment seeks to utilize the patient's unused potential. Improvement or refinement of old skills as well as development of new skills is usually possible in nearly all patients. Feldenkrais notes that the average human being uses less than 10 percent of their actual neurological potential.

When assessing the capabilities of the elderly, more than with any other group, it is most often impossible to presume anything about how a disease or group of diseases will affect the person's functional skills. The initial physical therapy assessment must determine if the foundation is established for using *active treatment* approaches or whether it is necessary to begin with *supportive therapeutic* approaches (Table 1-1). Traditional physical therapy treatment approaches have primarily been active and have made certain basic presumptions about the patient (see Table 1-1).

The average elderly patient being considered for a rehabilitation program cannot begin with a purely active treatment program. Such patients manifest at least one and often several of the characteristics which necessitate a supportive therapeutic approach as the point at which to start PT. The key to geriatric rehabilitation is to adapt the therapy to the real needs of the patient. A patient who is treated with a style of therapy suited to the needs of the moment can gradually benefit from the more active forms of therapy. Sup-

Table 1-1. Patient Characteristics and Physical Therapy Treatment

Treatment	
Active	Supportive
Patient motivated	Patient near burnout
Not in mourning	In mourning (justifiably depressed)
Emotional support	Limited emotional support
Minimal stress prior to current injury/problem	Stress symptoms (Urinary frequency, sleeping dysfunctions, high blood pressure, etc.)
Normal posture (plumb line)	Abnormal posture
Functional cardiopulmonary system	Limited endurance
Will power learning	Subconscious learning

portive physical therapy that may be used initially with a depressed or very ill patient can include heat, massage, breathing facilitation, positioning, Feldenkrais functional integration, etc. The basic criteria for a supportive physical therapy approach is that the patient should be able to experience a physiological/functional benefit without being highly motivated, with or without using concentration, will power, and effort; it should feel pleasant to the patient. The initial goal of a supportive physical therapy approach is to: (1) build a bond of trust; (2) decrease unnecessary stress; (3) at the same time, facilitate relaxation; and (4) facilitate normalization of breathing and ease of movement in all the noninvolved areas of the body (maximize the total functional ability of all aspects of the person not directly injured or diseased). Thus, the goal of supportive PT is to reduce and eliminate all unnecessary splinting and adaptive postures/functions, which are not seen as desirable. The use of supportive PT techniques allows the rehabilitation team to obtain a truer picture of the elderly client's potential for improvement. The most important aspect of the initial use of supportive forms of PT is the motivational value and the positive impact it usually has on building the bond of trust.

The development of new skills using both supportive and active PT approaches begins the moment the therapist and the patient meet. As the patient begins to master a new skill, the process of *skill transference* must be initiated in many cases. First, under the supervision of the PT, the patient must be encouraged to practice the skill in the natural setting where it is to be used (bedroom, bathroom, etc.). The personnel on the nursing unit then must be taught how to guard as needed and to cue to help the patient under the active supervision of the PT. Next, the primary nurse or caregiver and the patient carry out the entire skill with the PT observing from a distance. The PT will then need to recheck periodically and be available as a consultant. The patient should not walk only in physical therapy, remaining afraid to walk on the nursing unit with nursing personnel. The skill development must include a program for active carryover into the patient's real life. A stable skill becomes a part of the restorative nursing plan of care, and these improvements in functional ability improve the patient's self-confidence, gradually strengthening the role of the nurse as a teacher and an enabler making work with the patient easier in the long run.

CONCLUSION

The conceptual model for geriatric rehabilitation is an itemized checklist designed for the members of the rehabilitation team. The physical therapist's actual treatment contribution rests solidly on effective organization of the initial steps of facilitating the growth of motivation and on effective implementation of a restorative nursing plan of care. As a contributing member in patient assessment, the physical therapist has a major responsibility for helping to itemize the patient's current functional skills (physical, social, emotional). Developing new and enhanced functional skills is most easily accomplished when it is not done at the expense of isolating the patient emotionally from family or friends. Geriatric rehabilitation is a process that requires attention to the details of human growth; first, the person needs to be groomed to their personal standard, dressed in their own clothes, fed, feeling safe and unafraid, and without urinary/bowel urgency. Then the patient is capable of focusing on how to learn a new functional skill. The details that make each of us feel like an individual are at least as important as our structural/muscular potential. The drive to live and to choose to participate comes from inside the person; that is the spark that must be lit if rehabilitation at any age is to succeed.

REFERENCES

1. Feldenkrais M: The Elusive Obvious. Meta Publications, California, 1981
2. Jackson O (ed): Physical Therapy of the Geriatric Patient. Churchill Livingstone, New York, 1983
3. Tallmer M (ed): The Life-Threatened Elderly. Columbia University Press, New York, 1984
4. Burchfield RW (ed): Oxford English Dictionary. Vol. H–N. Oxford at Clarendon Press, 1976
5. de Bono, E: New Think. Avon, New York, 1971
6. Murray RB, Huelskoetter MMW: Psychiatric Mental Health Nursing—Giving Emotional Care. Prentice-Hall, Englewood Cliffs, New Jersey, 1983
7. Murray RB: The person on the health-illness continuum: Promoting adaptation to the stress response. In Murray RB, Huelskoetter MMW: Psychiatric Mental Health Nursing–Giving Emotional Care. Prentice-Hall, Englewood Cliffs, New Jersey, 1983
8. Quinn JL: TRIAGE, An alternative approach to care for the elderly, 1974–1979. Connecticut Department on Aging, Hartford, Connecticut, 1980
9. Bandler R, Grinder J: Frogs into Princes, Neurolinguistic Programming. Real People Press, Moab, Utah, 1979
10. Weston L: Body Rhythm: The Circadian Rhythms Within You. Harcourt Brace Jovanovich, New York, 1979
11. Jackson O: Brain function, aging and dementia. In Umphred D (ed): Neurological Rehabilitation, Mosby Co., St. Louis, 1984

2 | Learning Strategies: A Communications Model

Elizabeth Dickinson

"What about growing old upsets you?"

"Because you stop learning."

"Why does that upset you?"

"Because if you stop learning, why live?"

"Then, are you saying that living is learning?"

"Yeah, maybe. Or learning is living."

"Do you believe that?"

"Yes."

"Then what about growing old upsets you?"

"You stop learning."

"Do you believe that?"

This is a question too often answered from a cultural bias. Possibly we can afford to have sexual and religious biases, but to discriminate against growing older is something none of us can afford to do. We grow older from the moment we are born. But we are now realizing, with scientific evidence that how we grow old may be a learned response.

Do you believe that?

Let me tell you a story, a true story.*

METAPHORS

The telephone rang. A voice on the other end said in a clear, efficient tone, "Your father is getting senile." My brothers and I had just placed our parents in a nursing home, at their request. My parents could no longer care for each

---

* This chapter is based on NLP, (neurolinguistic programming) strategies. It is intended to provide a personal experience in the ease of communication.

other's health needs and did not want to be dependent on their children, yet they wanted to continue a life together. A nursing home had seemed to be the answer. What had gone wrong? Instead of asking that question, I immediately internalized my emotions and felt guilty. I was no better than all the other children who "put" their parents in nursing homes. But worse than that, I had lost the father whose wisdom I had depended on all my life. How could he do this to me—become senile? The voice on the other end interrupted my internal dialogue. "The doctors would like to set up a meeting with you. Can you come as soon as possible?" I answered that I could come right away. The person on the other end hung up. I was left with a dead phone receiver clamped to my ear. What I knew was that I did not want to see the doctors. They could not answer my questions. I wanted to see my father not someone labeled senile.

I sat on the edge of his bed. He sat opposite me in the lounge chair we had purchased to celebrate his arrival at the nursing home, holding his empty pipe cupped in the palm of his hand, complying with the nursing home rules forbidding smoking. I wanted to cry. He was the father who used to make me laugh, but with his head hanging he resembled the image of a senile old man.

"Dad." I asked, "how did you get senile?" I blurted it out like the two-year-old asking for his wisdom, as if asking, "How does the sun get up in the morning?" He half rose from his chair, fell back, and we all held our breath. It was my mother in her matching lounge rocker who returned us to reality.

"Ellis," my mom called to him. Her voice was calm. He did not rise from the chair but his blood pulsed visibly in the vein at the top of his skull.

"Maybe they're right," he said.

"What can't you do?" I asked. I was not talking to someone senile; nor was I talking to my dad when I was two years old asking him to solve the problems of the world. My own adult mind had returned, asking for information.

"I can't remember those damn doctors' names. They're all foreigners." This statement was not due to prejudice. My father was a curious man and always celebrated getting to know someone who was different as an opportunity for new learning.

"What about their being foreign bothers you?" I asked.

"I can't remember their names."

"I'll be right back," I said. I went to the nurse's station and asked for a list of the doctors' names.

"We're sorry," the nurse on duty said. "We didn't know you would be here so soon. We would have called the doctors to set up a meeting."

"I don't think that will be necessary," I said. "I just want the list of names." The nurse shrugged her shoulders. She obviously could see no reason for it, but she complied. I returned with the list of names—Indian names for the most part, three of them—to my father's room and again sat on the edge of the bed. I spelled each name for him. He saw the spelling and pronounced the name, names I could not pronounce not having heard them; now he was able to match the word he saw in his mind with the pronunciation he remembered hearing. He had it.

Table 2-1. Representational Images, Symbols, and Associated Physiological, Voice and Breathing Characteristics and Common Predicates

Symbol	Image		Eye Position	Body Posture	Voice Tone	Breathing	Predicates
	Nature	Kind					
V^c V_r V	Visual	Constructed Remembered Undetermined	Up {Right {Left Defocused	— Erect —	— High —	— In upper chest —	Appear, observe, cloudy, watch, look, draw, image, glance, see, show, clear, dark, light, pattern, etc., A color, a shape, a size
A_c A_r A_{id}	Auditory	Constructed Remembered Self-discussion	Level {Right {Left {Left Down	— Intermediate Chin in hand	— Midrange —	— In diaphragm —	Music, tempo, clang, ring, discuss, whisper, clatter, talk, speak, sing, tone, noise, loud, soft, voice, call, tell, listen, etc.
K	Kinesthetic	Undetermined	{Right	Slumped	Low	In stomach area	Feel, hurt, lift, tender, reach, take, firm, soft, push, sturdy, stiff, run, handle, catch, hold, etc.
Unspecified predicates	—	—	—	—	—	—	Seem, have, think, allow, believe, aware, must, do, want, shall, know, sense, understand, make, be, etc.

i, internal; d, digital.
I wish to acknowledge Leslie Cameron-Bandler, one of the cofounders of the NLP model, for the development of this chart and also for her encouragement of my work in integrating the NLP model and the Feldenkrais work.

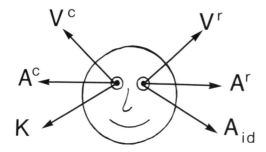

Fig. 2-1. Symbols represent characteristic associated eye position during thought processing. Abbreviations for symbols as in Table 2-1.

"I'm not as fast a learner as I once was," he said, laughing at himself, "but with practice I might improve."

"Now, Ellis," my mom said, and they smiled at each other. They were "at home" now and so was I, responding to the familiar tones of their voices and the smiles on their faces.

What I knew about my father was that his preferred learning mode was *visual*, despite his focal blindness. Although we all have available the various learning modes—visual, auditory, kinesthetic, olfactory, and gustatory—we usually have one favorite mode to represent in consciousness what we know (See Fig. 2-1 and Table 2-1). In his active living, my father was a brilliant mathematician. He could see all the pages of a textbook in his mind's eye. In later years, when his own eyesight failed him, my mother would read aloud, becoming his eyes. He would continue making internal pictures to match her words, because he knew the figures, symbols, and words. He had actually seen them before. The doctors' names were words he had never seen, and he could not make internal pictures to match the words. Once I spelled them for him, he saw them and could match them to the information he had stored, albeit unconsciously at the time, in his auditory memory. And, in truth, if he had more practice in "learning" he might well resume his speed.

How often do patients in a nursing home get to practice their learning skills? Practice of skills require three things: curiosity, knowledge of how a person learns, and a change in our belief systems about the elderly. This change in belief systems depends on what we believe about ourselves.

"Then what about growing old upsets you?"

"You can't learn."

Do you believe that? If your answer is no, we can continue. If it is yes, you may wish to continue solely out of curiosity.

NEUROLINGUISTIC PROGRAMMING

To gather information as to why my father was not learning I used a model based on neurolinguistic programming (NLP) (see Table 2-1). The model recognizes the fact that we receive information through our five senses (V, visual; A, auditory; K, kinesthetic; G, gustatory; O, olfactory). Using the same senses, we process the information (in other words, think) and store it (memory, to be recalled later). We use these same sensory modalities to represent the information in our consciousness when we act. Although each person has all modes available in the unconscious (V,A,K,G,O), the mode we choose for conscious representation determines how we know what we know and is what allows us to act on that knowing.

My father's favorite mode for knowing is his visual system. He has access to his other modes if he is led to them, as he demonstrated when he "remembered" the auditory pronunciation of his doctors' names once he saw them spelled on his internal visual screen. In NLP, we refer to this process of leading as crossing representational systems or cross-repping. It is a technique for increasing our flexibility and a technique I often use in consulting with students at the university. Why not use cross-repping with an elderly patient? I am speaking specifically of learning strategies with the elderly, so why not use a good learning technique any time and any place?

Another NLP technique makes use of "anchors." The NLP model assumes that all the information received, whether from internal or external sources, is stored, and that information received is simultaneously linked, whether consciously or unconsciously, in all modalities (V,A,K,G,O). Recalling one modality triggers the recall of the original simultaneous linking. For example, many of us have developed a conscious strategy for remembering in which we link an item to be recalled to another item, such as a name to a face. The trick is to find a connector, or what we call anchor, for remembering, such as a familiar touch, a particular tone of voice, or a visual image. But anchors are much more than tools useful for recall of information. They are keys to unlocking the complex and wonderful human mind/body system, a system more sophisticated than any computer storage and retrieval feedback/feedforward loop yet imagined. An anchor can induce a complete physiological state.

Suppose I go home and press the switch to hear the messages recorded on my telephone answering machine. A single word, spoken in a certain tone, can induce a physiological state that could be detected by electrodes placed on my skin, and an astute observer could notice the muscles of my face change, flatten, and relax, along with a defocusing of my eyes, a dilation of my pupils, perhaps an intake of breath—a readiness for hearing word content, a physiology for learning (as we might call it in an academic setting). Such physiological states are now being studied and researched for their impact on learning. Learning and teaching are basically processes of good communication. Therefore, why not make use of such research any place and any time when we want to communicate and get our message across.

Another equally familiar example, is the experience of a voice tone that elicits a tightening of the muscles, a drop in temperature of the skin, a holding of the breath—that is, a posture of defense. No longer can we hear the content of the message as we are overwhelmed by the trigger or anchor to the physiological state of fear, insecurity, or even anger. If we want to learn, hear, or see, the anxiety state is not useful. We must change our anchors, regain control of our world for new choices, *access a state of self confidence, which is a physiological state for learning*. But the elderly who have become "patients" are not aware of their anchors, nor are we, the caretakers, aware of triggering them. Such awareness is two-sided, with us as persons who are growing older and with us as caretakers—still, the same person.

The Physiology of Learning

"Now, Ellis," my mom said, as if they were at home. Being at home is a positive, physiological state, a state for learning that mother has triggered with her voice tone, her smile, and anchor. If we are not physically at home, we can take our anchors with us. My mother and father were anchors for each other. However, with appropriate anchors, we can be at home with anyone, smiling back to a fellow rider on a bus who smiles our way is an anchor for a pleasant physiological state. Politeness is not simply a "should"; it is respect for "the other" and a very useful and powerful anchor.

"Let's go for a smoke," my father says. He has his pipe in hand and a grin on his face. "One of the rules," he says. It is a rule my brothers and I thought he would never accept, considering his pipe as much a part of him as his breath. In the nursing home, he was not allowed to smoke in his room but had to go to the smoking room.

"Turn left," he directs me, just in time before I turned right. "Second door," he says, and he is smiling with his almost blind eyes on the horizon, seeing pictures in his mind of the path for his feet. New rules are new learning, and those entering an institutional setting (temporary or permanent) may have more to learn at a faster pace than at any other time since childhood. Most of us as little children were respected and allowed to learn how to walk, how to talk, and how to be in this world easily and at our own rates. The comfortable, at home anchored learning was probably the fastest and the most competent understanding we have ever achieved and certainly the most complicated. Do we lose that ability to learn?

Neurolinguistic programming offers us a technique for discovering how we learn, reconnecting us to the physiology of learning. We look up with our eyes when we are making pictures, look right and left of mid-body when we are hearing words or composing our own words, look down left for talking to ourselves and down right to access our feeling state. This is a description of typical right-handed wiring, although some left-handed persons may function in reverse fashion. Our words match this wiring, the predicates of what we use. The person who says, "I see what you are saying" is doing just that, seeing internal pictures which he believes represent your meaning. The person who says, "It sounds good to me" actually hears it sound that way, in so many words. Do you, the reader, follow me now? Or are you "in touch" with what I am saying? If you were to monitor your body carefully enough, you could identify the feeling in your body that lets you know the answer to my question. We are often aware of our negative feedback: 5 times 8 is not 45. (How do you know that it's not?) The positive feeling often proceeds from our awareness although it is essential for the necessary flexibility for new learning. To feel good, or the extent to which you make yourself feel good, could be an IQ measure in a nursing home as well as in a university. The body–mind system is a curious critter, and we can be curious in all representational systems, the sensory-motor complexes representing what we are aware of; usually pictures, words, sounds, and feelings.

But what about the senses of smell and taste? These senses can provide powerful anchors, not as useful in a university setting as in a hospital or nursing home. Let me tell you another story. I was again visiting my parents in the "living room" of their nursing home. I was walking down the hallway when one of the "inmates" (as my father referred to himself and the others) reached out and grabbed me by the skirt from her lower position in a wheelchair.

"You smell like my red dress," she says, gripping the material of my blue skirt to her nose, holding me there as if we were in a Siamese embrace, a caricature tableau. There was no way I was going to get loose. My first impulse was to shout out for help, bringing one of the east-wing orderlies to cut me loose and return his charge to her cell or. . . .

"I had a red dress once," I said, talking more to myself than to her. I'm not sure it smelled like this one." Still talking to myself, I was bending down almost nose to nose with the lady from the east wing. She had not released me from her grip but she was smiling, seeing me.

"Mine had lace on it," she says.

"Mine, I think, was more rose than red," I say. We are talking to each other now.

"At the collar," she says and reaches up to my neck, letting go of the skirt. She runs her hand around my neck, circling it like a necklace with light delicate fingers. "I used to wear it to tea," she says. "Do you want to come to tea?" she asks me, her child-voice asking me to come to a tea party and bring my dolls.

"I can't today," I say. "I'm visiting my mother. Maybe another time."

"Oh, that's nice," she says. I think to myself that what is nice is that someday I will come to tea in her make-believe world. Her eyes are completely focused on me. "It's good to visit your mother," she says. She not only sees me now, she hears me. We are in rapport, a term we use in NLP to describe a normal process for communicating, but in the case of my friend at the nursing home, it first appeared to be abnormal and was labeled so by the staff as "out-to-lunch,"—just as my father was labeled senile. When this occurs, we contact a label rather than the real person behind the label. It is we, then, who could be labeled as out-to-lunch or "into labels." The friend that I had just made was not so much out-to-lunch as she was "into tea," in her own private world, which she chose, consciously or unconsciously, as a better place to be than in the nursing home. I joined her in her world.

I have a lot of questions to ask her now. Is she a mother? Does she have children? Do they visit her? But a nurse comes along and wheels her away at breakneck speed. She doesn't look back.

Most people in our culture have a model of the world quite similar to ours;

we call that model reality, and we call those people normal. We do not have to enter each other's world consciously in order to communicate. With the elderly, especially those who have suddenly been displaced into an institution (hospital or nursing home) it may take a conscious effort not to talk down to them or even to pretend but to use our senses to see and hear what they are saying instead of going inside ourselves—into the labels of our learning—and labeling them and then contacting them as labels.

Each of us has our own internal and external worlds. Going in and out of these worlds is the road we travel in our daily working and personal lives. At times the external world is emphasized more, particularly in our career-centered life or when raising our children; but when we become elderly, the external world ceases to have the choices it once did, and we choose to spend more time in our internal processes of remembering or pretending, if we are lucky. My friend in the wheelchair had not given up her desire to make contact with the external world, as some do. She had invited me in, reached out to me, grabbed my skirt, so strong was her desire. If I had yanked away or thought her crazy, or had been frightened by her grip on my skirt, I would have missed meeting someone new. I would also have missed meeting a part of myself and an opportunity to learn. But most important, I would have missed the opportunity *to lead her back into "reality,"* the reality of where she was in the present here-and-now.

On the next visit to the nursing home, I saw her sitting in her wheelchair in the corner of the entrance lobby. I waved to her and she waved back. We went for a walk, side by side, she in her wheelchair, me on my feet, my hand pushing her wheelchair at the pace she might have walked if she had been walking, not riding, a pace a little slower than my own. We had a conversation about all the questions I wanted to ask, and then she said that it looked like a nice spring day outside.

In NLP, the process we had just experienced is called pacing and leading. Once we have met another person in his or her model of the world, we can lead them to ours. We have a responsibility, then, for the model of our world, that it be a good one so that they may want to stay, or they will return to their private "tea-parties." How do we make nursing homes, or any environment, a good place to be when we get older?

In our culture, the environment is a deprived one for the elderly. There is not much to do that seems worthwhile. Elderly persons, if they are smart at all, enter their internal world and are fortunate if they have nice tea parties to go to there. The loss may not be so much that of the elderly as ours. We have lost them by treating them as labels.

I lose my father when I think of him as senile; the doctor loses his patient; the teacher loses her student. Labels are abstractions, descriptions and, as such, can be useful tools for certain kinds of communication. But when the verbs, or verbals of description, become nouns like tables and chairs, we had better look again. In NLP, we test "real" nouns by asking the question, "Can I carry it in a wheelbarrow?" Perhaps I could carry my father, but not "senility." Returning a noun, or a nominative, to a verb, gives us back our freedom, our consciousness of abstracting, our senses for seeing and hearing and feeling. I am describing a communication model, and as long as we live with another person on this planet, the challenge of communication is with us. It is impossible for us to communicate without doing so both verbally and nonverbally, and the response we elicit is what we communicate. If someone acts senile, what are we communicating? If we want another response, we must change our communication. The flexibility is our own power. What did we really mean to say?

Curiosity

To answer the question of what we really meant to say we must separate our intention from our communication—do we intend to talk to a "senile person" or to a person with a difficulty? What is the outcome we intend? My father had difficulty remembering his doctors' names. The intended outcome was to help him remember. The method by which the intention is achieved is the challenge of our work motivated by our own curiosity. A beloved teacher of mine, Moshe Feldenkrais, told his students over a cup of coffee that the sense that made the difference between humans and non-humans was a sense of curiosity. The problem of growing old is not so much sitting on porches in rocking chairs, or even sitting in wheelchairs in nursing homes, but sitting without curiosity.

If we separate our intention from our communication (do we intend to talk to a senile person or to a person with a difficulty wanting to solve that difficulty?) how do we communicate to get the response we want? What response do we want? Do we want the person to act like a senile person, confirming our diagnosis? We must look at our intended outcome. Is it based on external awareness of internal diagnosis? We all travel from external to internal worlds. As long as we are in the mainstream of making a living and raising a family, the external world is more dominant. But age gives us time to indulge our internal sense, to sit on porches in rocking chairs, to stare out at the world as we visit the past, or hold grandchildren on our laps and tell them stories from the past. Now we place ourselves in nursing homes and tell stories to ourselves. Sometimes we talk out loud so we can better hear ourselves. Our internal reality takes precedence over the external reality. Which world is reality, then, becomes a judgment.

Aging and Thinking

Aging has been thought to be a downhill process, a one-way street into neurological and functional loss, a degenerative process. But we are beginning to see that this process does not have to occur. We have facts to the contrary, that neurons have the capacity to form new dendritic and axonal material as well as new synapses and that thinking itself is a physiological process. That we are what we think we are is more than a platitude.

When you look up, make a picture of who you think you are, step into that picture, and have the feeling of being that person, you are creating your own physiology. This process continues unconsciously based on our belief systems. Change our belief systems and we change the outcomes. Change what we say to ourselves and our pictures change. Perhaps we all need to talk out loud so that we can hear outselves better. The understanding of the computer age has also brought us an understanding of how our brains create their own software. A great difference between computers and their artificial intelligence and our brains is the answer to the question: Who is doing the programming?

THE FELDENKRAIS METHOD

The interface between the Feldenkrais method and NLP creates the possibility of answering this question with the words, "I am." The Feldenkrais method is a physiological approach (which is not the province of this chapter but is discussed in other chapters) to the flexibility of our primary learning, our first learning—rolling over, sitting, standing, and knowing who we are: NLP is a physiological approach to what might be called our secondary learning—how we represent in consciousness who we are. *You can perform "physical therapy" with words as well as with your hands.* In the best of models, the two approaches are not separate. I have seen Dr. Feldenkrais teach a lesson, never putting his hands directly on the person. But the person looked up, saw what Dr. Feldenkrais was saying, and changed from a posture of depression (eyes down, body down, slumped in wheelchair) to a flexibility of movement, able to look up, right and left, as well as down. But sometimes unable to sustain this posture, owing to the "environment" of the wheelchair, built for slumping and looking down, the patient often, inadvertently, became depressed again. Secondary experiences are often based on primary sensations. Depressions, paranoia, even schizophrenia, are responses to the communication of our environments, (ie, furniture as well as people); so are elation, contentment, and reality. Return the nouns to verbs, and we may be able to find out what is depressing our client, making our client senile. Labels are no more than disguised verbs. In NLP, we say, "Labels cannot be carried in a wheelbarrow, no matter how large the wheelbarrow." So get them out of the wheelbarrow, or wheelchair, and put them back on their feet or their seats so that they can move in order to learn.

"What about growing old upsets you?"

When my father said he could not remember the names of his doctor, his eyes were looking up left but there was nothing there. He could not see internally what he had not seen externally, and his eyes went down right and stayed there, along with his body. When I spelled the words, the names of his doctors flashed like neon signs in his internal screen, bringing him, quite literally, up and into this world. When the woman greeted me as if I were herself in her little red dress with the lace collar, her eyes were down right, smelling the fabric of my blue skirt which was red in her mind. *I did not correct her because I would have been wrong.* The picture in her mind had a little red dress in it, not a blue skirt. We call her "crazy," but who is the crazy one, the person reacting to a picture in his head or the person reacting to a label in his head? We see that label instead of the person.

I would much rather be writing this chapter about the elderly for the elderly, not for the physical therapist or the doctor or the nurse, except that the physical therapist, doctor, and nurse will also become the elderly. So what must change is our own attitude toward ourselves, right now before we get elderly, and that too is a label.

BELIEF SYSTEMS

Recently, I took my two granddaughters to visit their great grandmother, whom they call "big grandma" from their perspective of looking up at her in her magnificent throne of a wheelchair that moves without legs. My granddaughters are two and four years old. On the way home, from the backseat of the car, the four-year-old's voice piped into my ear whispering a secret.

"Nana," she asked, "when I get old like big grandma, can I live in a nursing home?" I did not ask what picture she was making in her head, but it was different from the one in most of our heads. She might have been asking if she could live in a dorm when she goes away to college.

"Me, too," said the two-year-old, wanting what she did not even know, not overhearing our secret. It is not our attitude toward nursing homes that must change, or even our attitude toward the elderly, but our attitude toward ourselves, even at the age of two or four. That is the beginning of getting old.

"Yes," I said, "if you want to." And I prayed silently for their *right to want to or not* when they were as old as their "big grandma." But it's not a prayer that will make the difference. It's our belief system.

"Then what about growing old upsets you?"

SUGGESTED READINGS

Neurolinguistic Programming

Bandler R, Grinder J: Frogs Into Princes. Real People Press, Moab, Utah, 1979

Cameron-Bandler L: They Lived Happily Ever After. Meta Publication, Lake Oswego, OR, 1978

Dilts R: Roots of Neuro-Linguistic Programming. Meta Publications, Lake Oswego, OR, 1983

Dilts R: Applications of Neuro-Linguistic Programming. Meta Publications, Lake Oswego, OR, 1983

Gordon D: Therapeutic Metaphors. Meta Publications, Lake Oswego, New York, 1978

The Feldenkrais Method

Feldenkrais M: Body and Mature Behavior. International Universities Press, New York, 1949

Feldenkrais, M: Awareness Through Movement. Harper and Row, New York, 1972

Feldenkrais, M: The Elusive Obvious. Meta Publications, Lake Oswego, OR, 1981

Belief Systems

Bandler R: Frogs Into Princes. Real People Press, Moab, Utah, 1979

Jackson O: *Brain functions, Aging and dementia.* In Neurological Rehabilitation. CV Mosby, St Louis, 1984

Kaufman B: To Love is to Be Happy With. Fawcett Crest Books, New York, 1977

Wheatley D: Editorial. Stress Med 1985; 1:157

3 | Facilitating Movement: A Conceptual Model

Darcy Umphred
Gordon Burton

MUTUAL RESPECT

I look to you, your body flexed
Your eyes stare at the floor.
Will you share your inner world
To this stranger at the door?

The door is not a sided frame
But a wall between two shells.
One is mine, the other yours
Can we touch those inner wells?

You have so much to teach to me
And I to share with you.
We now must shed our fears of age
And search for what is true.

You are a person just as I
With pain and joy to feel
Please share those inner insights.
Your wisdom to reveal.

And I as friend can walk with you
As strength along your side
Today please stand with head held high
There is no need to hide.

D.A.U.
June 14, 1985

Childhood, adolescence, young adulthood, middle age, and geriatrics, all represent sequential stages in the development of humans. Early stages of life are represented by steady change in distinct movement patterns and attitudes toward the environment and myelination or functioning of the central nervous system (CNS). Geriatrics is not different. In order to understand fully and work effectively with aged persons, one can develop a conceptual model. This model should not differentiate these people from the total framework of the development of humans. Instead, it should identify features that may make this group of people unique. This model and the understanding of age-related characteristics should help the physical therapist, occupational therapist, and other health professionals deal comfortably and with optimal sensitivity when interacting with the elderly. The primary focus of this chapter is the presentation of such a conceptual model.

Most health professionals dealing with problems encountered by the elderly are not aged themselves. Thus, collegial understanding of the problems encountered by older people is vicarious and theoretical. For this reason, a sensitivity and a willingness to learn from our elderly clients without prebiasing our opinion or belief seems paramount if obtaining optimal physical and emotional integration is a treatment goal. A conceptual model can help health professionals grasp a sense of the multidimensional characteristics of each human being. Yet a model can only give a sense of the whole. Each client is an individual with unique experiences, different learning styles, varied likes and dislikes, degrees of motivation, and acceptance of independence. Each adult's individuality must not only be identified and accepted but must also be allowed to continue developing. Often, as young and middle-aged professionals, we categorize the elderly into groups. The more we categorize and label the aged population, the more we insulate ourselves from the shocking reality that this at some time will be us. We protect ourselves by creating "conceptualizations" that make the elderly, by definition, different from us. We can then use terms, labels, and categorizations which allow "objectivity." We must reduce our distance and acknowledge our fears before we can reach out to the geriatric person and build a trusting relationship between us. Then, instead of forcing an activity, we must allow the elderly adult to choose the direction of growth that best meets his or her personal needs.

BASIC CONCEPTUAL MODEL

The brain is a logical organism and as such is organized to progress with optimal efficiency. At least three major topic areas can be analyzed when the function of the CNS is discussed.

First, the behavioral responses of humans reflect processing of input from past memory and present input modalities as well as functioning of the motor control system itself. *Second*, the innate structures and function of the human CNS gives important data regarding potential therapeutic intervention and its likelihood for success. *Third*, the individual learning styles and environmental experiences of each elderly person have direct impact on the creation of an optimal learning experience conducive to her or his needs and choices. Figure

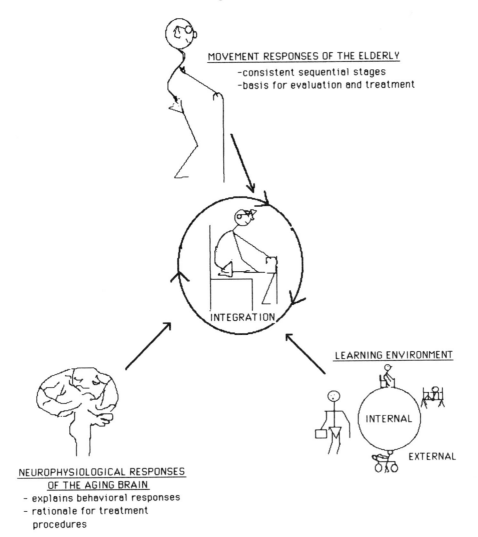

MOVEMENT RESPONSES OF THE ELDERLY
-consistent sequential stages
-basis for evaluation and treatment

INTEGRATION

LEARNING ENVIRONMENT

INTERNAL

EXTERNAL

NEUROPHYSIOLOGICAL RESPONSES
OF THE AGING BRAIN
- explains behavioral responses
- rationale for treatment
  procedures

Fig. 3-1. Conceptual Model: Clinical triad—categories of factors involved in a treatment process.

3-1 illustrates the interrelationship of these three conceptual categories as a clinical triad.

MOVEMENT RESPONSES OF THE ELDERLY

The range of potential movement responses observed in the child and the young adult are more global than those observed in the elderly. What is normal for an adolescent may not be normal for a 70-year-old person. Similarly, what is normal at 92 years of age may be considered abnormal at 21 years of age. For example, a slight unintentional tremor in a young adult would be considered a potential hard-core neurological sign of basal ganglia problems, although the same tremor in an 85-year-old person would be considered merely a symptom of old age and not alarming. Understanding the behavioral differences between youth, middle age, and geriatrics should help the clinician set realistic expectations for alternative movement responses for any age group. This knowledge of behavioral responses should directly influence treatment programs. The flexed posture that leads to hip and knee flexion contractures, kyphosis, rounded shoulders, and forward head posturing in an older person should inform the therapist that this person cannot lie comfortably in a prone position. Although the therapist may have learned that the prone position is excellent for some treatment goal, it may be a totally unrealistic position for an older client. This is only one of the many examples illustrating the need for behavioral assessment of the client's ability based on his or her repertoire of responses at a specific time. The client's existing potential for behavioral responses should guide the direction of assessment and treatment intervention.

Prior to establishing goals and treatment sequences, the therapist must evaluate the client's motor skill level. No matter what assessment tool is used, results are based on the individual's motoric ability to accomplish an identified task. The patient response required may be gross or fine motor skill of the hand, mouth, or eye; it may even be a lack of response. Usually, clinicians address problem areas in which a client cannot perform. Often on the assumption that repetition will lead to motor skill and control over behavioral responses, treatment consists of repetitive exercises or opportunities for the elderly client to practice the desired behavior. If, instead of addressing the activities the client cannot accomplish successfully, therapists analyze those responses in which the elderly person is successful, and why the person is successful, a better assessment of the functional potential and the status of the older individual's CNS can be obtained.

What the client can do is a direct reflection of CNS processing. Failure to perform tells the clinician that something is wrong but in no way explains where the problems exist. For example, observing a successful bed-to-chair transfer gives the clinician important data about range of motion, muscle strength, reflexology, balance or equilibrium responses, verticality, body schema and position in space, spatial relationships, motor planning, and sequential processing. Determining whether the client was asked, visually shown, or kinesthetically guided through the activity helps the therapist assess sensory input and processing. When a client then fails at a tub transfer, the therapist has a much better idea of the reason for the lack of success. Many components of a bed-to-chair transfer are also incorporated in a chair-to-tub movement pattern. That is, activities of daily living (ADL) assessments are sequentially based on the difficulty of the task. The ADL tasks tested initially are foundation patterns incorporated into movement sequences tested in more complex tasks. Being able to identify what is similar and what is different helps establish those specific areas in which the client has difficulties. By focusing therapy on either direct intervention or alternative behavioral responses, the clinician can more clearly focus treatment sequencing, thus reducing frustration for both the client and the clinician.

Once an elderly person's functional ability has been evaluated, appropriate goal setting and treatment planning can more realistically be established. In order for the therapeutic interventions to be successful, they must be based on an understanding of the existing behavioral responses controlled by the CNS, the person's potential repertoire of movement patterns, any additional physical or emotional limitations (orthopedic, cardiac, or respiratory), and the normal effect of the aging process on CNS function.

Symptoms that are acceptable in the elderly client may not be appropriate in a younger person. Our norms and expectations must be compatible with age-appropriate responses. Many behaviors are learned; equally, some failures are accepted as we mature to old age. Similarly, an understanding of normal aging and of ways in which a person may compensate behaviorally for a normal degenerating input (vision changes), processing difficulties, or motor control system disturbances helps the therapist distinguish between what is truly an acute problem and what are chronic problems that are now observable due to a loss in the compensatory system. For example, an elderly person who has suffered a stroke with resulting hemianopsia may demonstrate severe loss of proprioceptive-vestibular awareness. This observable deficit may have been owing to a chronic, long-term degeneration of these two systems. The visual system may have compensated for the degenerative loss, with the client having no apparent deficit. Following the stroke, the client's visual system is affected, eliminating the compensatory mechanism. A therapist who assumes that the proprioceptive-vestibular loss results primarily from the acute CNS insult will expect spontaneous return or quick relearning for the client. Unrealistic goal setting would thus result, leading to failure on the part of both the therapist and client. We as therapists must allow our clients to teach us what they can and cannot do, what they desire and do not desire to do, and what they are motivated to work toward.

Behavior analysis of common movement distortions in the elderly not only assists in evaluation and goal setting, but also directs treatment sequencing. When limitations in the elderly population are considered, specific types of movements become identifiable. Postural function, rotatory patterns, reciprocal movements, quick equilibrium, and protective responses are major areas of motor impairment in many elderly persons. Lack of good postural extension patterns lead to a flexed body posture as well as an inability to maintain upright postures for long periods of time. The resultant fatigue leads to more frequent and longer periods of sitting, ending in an increase of flexion patterns and perpetuation of the cycle, further encouraging this rounded posturing. Posture and equilibrium are intimately connected. As a person loses postural function, sits more frequently and longer, does not challenge the balancing mechanism, these equilibrium responses also begin to shut down, making the person more apprehensive about moving except when necessary and thus encouraging more sitting. The lack of rotatory patterns leads to difficulty in turning to get out of bed, getting in and out of cars, cleaning the house, getting dressed, and controlling and modifying complex movement patterns. The elderly begin to engage in very symmetrical activities, such as log-rolling to turn over in bed, moving symmetrically in coming to a sitting position from a supine position, and in coming to a standing position from a sitting position, walking with little if any arm swing, decreasing social and sports activities, etc. In all movements, from the very basic to the very complex, the elderly person can be dramatically affected by lack of rotatory skills. Whether the decrease in function results from CNS degeneration due to aging or from disuse due to a reduced activity level, the result is another cycle of negative development in movement potential, leading to a very sedentary inflexible repertoire of motor responses which become increasingly difficult to reverse. Simultaneously, the fear of movement may be heightened if the client has had a friend who fell, broke a hip, went to a nursing home and, perhaps died.

In treating the elderly, we must ask whether these downward trends can be changed in order to increase mobility and freedom of movement within the elderly population. Anyone who works with the older adult can quickly answer yes as long as the client desires to improve. Creating treatment sequences that allow the client time to relearn at a pace conducive to his or her learning is critical. Similarly, determination of the components of a movement pattern that may be missing, such as rotation or postural function, and then helping the client relearn those components seems logical if carryover into other activities is desired.

The reasons for the loss by the elderly of specific components of motor responses and the best ways to facilitate relearning cannot be answered through behavioral analysis. Those unique features reflect the state of development of the client's entire body, mind, and experiences. Central nervous system function, cardiopulmonary ability, and orthopedic status must all be taken into consideration in order to comprehend fully the reasons for the behavior of the elderly person. Certain normal aging processes are occurring; they cannot be changed. Neither can the extent to which these changes are environmental rather than genetic be determined. By analyzing CNS function, a therapist can better comprehend why changes are occurring, where those aging processes will lead the elderly person, and how best to facilitate optimally through environmental input and prevent further deterioration. This concept leads to the second component of the model, neurophysiological responses of the aging brain.

NEUROPHYSIOLOGICAL RESPONSES OF THE AGING BRAIN

The science of brain functioning has advanced tremendously in the last 50 years. Today, humans still comprehend only a minute aspect of the function of brain processes. As our knowledge constantly advances, so does the state of any living brain a researcher or clinician may be studying. For this reason, colleagues working with the elderly must keep updating their understanding of neurophysiology and neuropsychology. Similarly, they must become keen visual and kinesthetic observers in order to keep abreast of the slight changes in motor responses that reflect brain changes in their clients.

Neurophysiology of Aging

Before a therapist can begin to comprehend the aged brain, an understanding of the functioning of the CNS before aging occurs is critical. Therapists treat clients by giving them input through one of a variety of sensory modalities in the hope that the client will make appropriate motor responses. Where each input system goes, how input is processed, and how to use specific treatment techniques in order to facilitate function optimally is not within the scope of this chapter. The reader may refer to additional studies.[1-3] With aging, some degeneration of the CNS occurs. Much has been written regarding neuromuscular and CNS changes with aging.[3] In 1931, Critchley made the first extensive investigation on changes with age, and his subsequent report which cited excellent descriptions of signs of disease and of pathology associated with old age, is a classic study of the neurology of the aged.[4] Although some question may remain regarding the exact degree of ongoing deterioration in the CNS, a reduction in the number of cells available to carry on normal CNS function cannot be denied. Although there is some evidence to suggest that the capillary network within the cortex is able to respond to changed metabolism and blood pressure[5], cellular atrophy has been shown to be complicated by diminished reserves of oxygen, protein, and tissue metabolism.[3,6-8] Definite changes occur within the CNS, including a weakening of facilitatory and inhibitory influences of higher centers within the brain over the lower centers.[9] Whether the changes within the brain effect intracentral or centroperipheral connections, they are an important factor in the alteration of the metabolic and overall functional control of the elderly and in the reduction of their adaptive abilities.

Changes in the peripheral nervous system and muscular system also materialize during the latter span of life. Although some neuromuscular changes are thought to be due to general deconditioning, changes also have been of a neurogenic origin.[3] Redistribution of muscle fibers or individual motor units indicates reinnervation due to sprouting of surviving neurons. This evidence supports the view that there is frequent denervation and reinnervation of limb and skeletal muscles in old age.[10]

Loss of general input or sensoriums also affect the person's normal feedback and compensatory mechanisms. Changes in normal visual acuity accommodation, ability to adapt to darkness, and degree of needed illumination are accepted problems of advanced age.[11] Changes in threshold of auditory perception also increase with age.[7,11] Tactile or cutaneous sensation decreases with age: sensory nerve endings are ~50 percent as numerous as they were at maturity.[12] Perception of vibratory sense is reported to increase in threshold by a significant degree.[7,13] Because of this relative sensory deprivation, the elderly client does not have normal feedback and compensatory mechanisms.[12]

Behavioral Implications

Understanding the physiological and neurological changes that occur with aging creates an opportunity to analyze the functional changes that so often are concurrent with aging. The concept of postural control implies intact connections between cortex, basal ganglia, and the vestibulocerebellar system, resulting in correct equilibrium in the standing posture. A disturbance of function anywhere along these pathways may give rise to difficulty in controlling body sway and create a genuine feeling of insecurity. Sheldon investigated the nature of the older person's loss of balance and increased tendency to fall. He concluded that the major cause of falls was a fundamental defect in the control of posture and gait. He also concluded that although there were some peripheral sensory abnormalities such as decreased proprioceptive and visual awareness, the primary problem was centrally oriented, particularly in the cerebellum, brain stem, and basal ganglia—the central control areas for posture and gait.[15] This study certainly helps a therapist understand why there is change with age in human walking patterns. General gait deviations with age include a decrease in stride length, an increase in stance phase-time ratio, a decrease in walking speed and increase in stride in the oldest groups, and a decrease in pelvic rotation.[16–18] Two additional changes in the cycle of gait, a greater excursion of total lateral displacement and an increase in the extension patterns and less flexion on the forward arc during arm swing, also occur.[13] (See Chapter 7 on gait changes with age for more detailed analysis). The muscles that show greatest loss of strength/coordination seem to be of the postural group: extensors of the neck, hip, and knee, abductors of the hip, and scapular and shoulder girdle stabilizers. That there is a physiological decline in strength/coordination together with increasing fatigability in the elderly is universally accepted. Although the changes occur in all muscle groups, they are most striking in the postural muscles, possibly accounting for the typical flexed posturing frequently seen in the geriatric client.

In light of the various studies regarding the CNS and neuromuscular systems, one may question the validity of evaluation results for clients suffering an acute onset of a CNS disorder. Our clients almost always have proximal, postural muscle involvement. Muscular return is often least evident in these muscle groups. Although we know that the lesion site has a dramatic effect on peripheral function, can we say that the functional clinical problem is due to the acute CNS disorder? Evaluation of equilibrium reactions can be similarly questioned.

Primitive postural reflexes in elderly subjects have also been reported[15] as has loss of higher center control over the brainstem area.[19] Loss of general muscle function and strength/coordination may lead to a problem in carrying out normal activities, placing additional stress on the elderly person. Healthy adults naturally call in compensatory systems to assist in gaining needed muscle tone when stress is present. Recruitment of tonic reflexes is evident in normal subjects.[20–22] Thus, an elderly person who needs more tone to perform a normal activity may consistently recruit those reflexes (increasing tone in flexors, adductors, and internal rotators). If the need is present and the reflexes are called into play, learning must be occurring. Many clients who seem to use tonic reflexes automatically following a CVA may have already learned those compensatory mechanisms. During treatment of the client, a therapist who wishes to inhibit these reflexes and facilitate higher center control may also have to consider memory and learning as processes that may also need modification.

Various changes in the nervous and muscular systems have been identified and their possible influence on normal adult activity mentioned.

Clinical Example

The changes that occur with old age may best be conceptualized if a specific problem observed in a client is discussed. Independent ambulation is usually considered a primary goal in working with a hemiplegic client. Energy expenditure is only one component of gait but is a factor certainly affected by age and may be very important when adaptations are considered in a treatment program. Loss of neuronal innervation; generalized weakness (especially of postural function), general decrease in tissue metabolism, protein binding, and oxygen saturation, loss of muscle fibers, and general decrease in normal balance have been connected to aging. After a CVA, even greater gait deviations, general loss of muscle function, and loss of adequate balance have been reported.[23,24] During independent ambulation without a brace or training device, a hemiplegic expends at least 100 percent more energy than is used in normal ambulation.[31] With training, all hemiplegics studied required at least 31 percent more energy than do normal subjects.[25,26] Hemiplegics require 40 to 50 percent more energy per step for walking up and down stairs.[27] If a client with a CVA requires more energy to perform activities yet has fewer resources, it is no wonder that both client and therapist often become frustrated. This problem certainly justifies setting normal movement patterns as a goal rather than encouraging abnormal patterns that not only increase energy consumption but often require bracing, which further increases energy demands. These investigators are not suggesting that certain treatment techniques are wrong or that bracing is never indicated; rather, we are advised to evaluate and reevaluate our goals and treatment procedures.

A therapist must always remember that the brain is organized to find efficient ways to respond to the world. If the response patterns of the elderly are perceived by us as distorted, inefficient, and in need of change, we must remember to evaluate the form of input/perception and response of the client since it may be the best available output pattern controlled volitionally by the client. To effect prolonged change in behavioral responses of a client, a therapist must first convince the client's "brain" (cognitive, emotional, and psychosocial beliefs) that the pattern is worth changing. Thus, analysis of reasons for a client's failure to perform will come from our understanding of behavioral sequencing and brain functioning. Intertwined, these two concepts give us a strong foundation for adaptation of treatment principles to meet the needs of the elderly. We have tended to regard the elderly as a group. Each client is a unique person with characteristics different from those of other unique elderly individuals. One must ask what resources the patient has with regard to sensory awareness, perceptual cognitive processing, emotional integrity, and motor control. These specific qualities must also be considered if a therapist intends to help the client meet specific personal needs. In other words, the therapist works and helps patients progress from where the patients are, not from where the therapist thinks they are. *To determine where patients are, verification that patients know where they are sensorially and what their bodies can do is critical.*

For example, assume that the therapist pushes on the foot of a patient who is resting supine, well-supported, and relaxed. The movement is started by gentle pressure under the heel, causing passive traction and approximation oscillations all the way up the body to the head. However, when asked, the patient responds that movement is felt up to the thigh only, sensing no movement above mid-thigh even though the therapist sees it. Obviously, the client's true perception is being distorted due to increased muscle tension, parietal lobe problems, internal capsule lesion, or some other neurologic problem. The treatment implication suggests that a therapist can only work from what the *patient can do* and *is aware of.* Asking the client to perform an ADL task that requires simultaneous awareness of the entire leg and trunk under stress is inappropriate. Increasing the sensory awareness of leg and trunk activities in less stressful and safer patterns should lead to better control and sequential progression to more neurologically advanced ADL tasks.

Discussion of each client's individual needs also focuses on the uniqueness of each patient as a learner. How learning and learning environments affect treatment sessions cannot be overemphasized and leads to the third component of the conceptual model.

LEARNING ENVIRONMENT

Although many clinicians have developed in-depth knowledge in the areas of sequential movement development (behavioral analysis) and the functioning of the CNS (neurophysiology and neuropsychology), what seems to make a clinician gifted is what people refer to as "the art of therapy." A few clinicians appear to have the talent the moment they enter the clinic; others, over time, seem to develop the skill; still many others strive but never obtain the gift. Response from clients to these few gifted clinicians seems magical and not limited to one client. Somehow these therapists seem to know what the patients need and then to help them find it. One critical characteristic of such gifted therapists is that they presume nothing about their client. They allow the client to be the initial teacher. With the bonding that occurs in such a relationship, both people learn from each other in a give-and-take interaction. As the patient directs and acts, the therapist assimilates the total and component responses in order to redirect, through input to the client, a new motor response that is more acceptable and efficient. This cycle of analysis–action–analysis is continual as long as the therapist and client are interacting in a therapeutic setting.

Gifted clinicians seem to know how to create a learning environment which optimally benefits the patient (they instantly adapt to the needs of the patient). For example, when regulating tone, an inexperienced clinician may have difficulty feeling tonal shifts. An inexperienced therapist feels and shifts neuromuscular function from too high to too low to slightly too high in a back-and-forth direction, having difficulty holding the tone steady as the noise in the room, the movement patterns, and multitudinous other stimuli keep altering the tone. The gifted therapist shifts the tone to a normal mode and maintains that tonal level no matter what external stimuli enter the client's input system.

Some therapists believe that a select few are born with an innate talent for clinical treatment; others believe that most people, with years of practice and supervision, can develop the skill and that a variety of learning strategies and sequences must be mastered, some of them as yet unknown. The more in-depth study clinicians pursue, the closer the art will match the science of therapy.

An important aspect of mastery of this art is an understanding of the environment in which it is practiced. An ice sculptor does not practice the art when the temperature is 105°F. Nor does an open-heart surgeon bring her team to the park for a change of scenery. Similarly, a therapist must match his skill to the environment in which he works. Some colleagues cannot work effectively with the elderly, others cannot work with middle-aged clients, and still others cannot work with children. Thus, the learning environment for both the client and the clinician plays a key role in the success or failure of any therapeutic intervention. In the totality of this environment, there are four subdivisions. First, the clients have an internal makeup that receives input, perceives input, processes it into an action, and responds to the input. Second, clients have an external world that controls the input to their internal systems. Therapists also have two environments. Thus, at any given moment of a learning interaction or therapy session, all four aspects of the whole must be considered (Fig. 3-2).

Client's Internal Environment

Preferential Learning Styles

The client's internal environment is the major focus of most therapists. What the client needs to learn and how to teach the client is commonly referred to as goal setting and treatment planning. Yet the client's internal world is very complex, and additional information is needed if we are to cause effective therapeutic changes and functional improvements. The elderly person has ex-

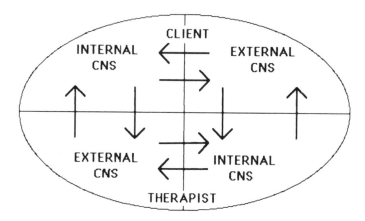

Fig. 3-2. Components of the learning environment.

perienced a maturation process that has helped to establish preferential learning styles. Vocational and recreational choices often reflect these learning strategies. A philosophy teacher must develop a high level of verbal strategies. An auto mechanic who can drop an engine, take it apart, put it together, and have it run perfectly, must have good visual–spatial skills. Very similar spatial skills are used by a sculptor, artist, or cartographer. A person's hobbies or recreational needs also reflect learning skills. Reading, skiing, photography, poetry writing, singing, and sky diving all have different characteristics that reflect processing in different areas of the brain.

If one enjoys processing input in one area and chooses not to engage in processing in another, preferential learning styles have been established. These styles are probably the most efficient for that person and, under stress, that person's brain makes choices reflecting those styles when trying to respond and control the external environment. Most normal adults have various ways in which they comfortably solve problems. As we get older, our preferential styles may become dominant and our ability to switch to alternative modes more limited. For that reason alone, it is important to determine through which input modality and which learning style an elderly client learns most efficiently. By creating an environment within which a client can optimally process, that person will feel less stress, accomplish more in a shorter time, and usually be more motivated to continue learning (see Chapter 2).

Normal Age-Related Changes and Learning

When the internal environment of the learner is considered, confounding variables regarding normal aging cannot be disregarded. Many clients enter a therapeutic setting following an acute medical insult such as a fractured hip, surgery, heart condition, or CVA. Normal changes with age have occurred irrespective of the acute problem. These changes, especially those within the limbic system, basal ganglia, and higher cortical regions, will dramatically affect a therapeutic interaction.

Psychomotor performance with respect to reaction time has consistently been identified as an age-related variable.[28–31] Older subjects require a longer preparatory interval between two successive stimuli, thus creating a decrease in reaction time.[32] No matter what the accepted rationale for the change in reaction time, the clinical sign persists. Normal changes with age decrease a person's ability to react to a single stimulus, let alone multistimuli of varying duration that are so often encountered in a clinical setting.

This general delay in response has also been reported in studies of memory. Older subjects always used more time regardless of difficulty with tests requiring retrieval of items related to short-term memory.[33] This time lag may be vital in any consideration of memory performance and forgetting. When the amount of recall needed is greater than the available retrieval time, obvious difficulty results. Older individuals have great difficulty in: (1) paced tasks, (2) tasks demanding constant switching of attention, and (3) tasks requiring frequent change of set.

All three areas are often identified as acute problems following a CNS insult.[33] This slowing of response time would certainly cause difficulty in interactions requiring immediate responses during a therapy session. Under time-pressured tasks, an elderly person's lack of ability to scan and retrieve rapidly as well as difficulty in reaction to several concomitant stimuli or serial stimuli would certainly affect scores on standardized cognitive, perceptual, and sensory motor tests. The total effect on the patient's sense of mastery will have an impact on his or her self-image; this cannot be ignored. If retrieval time rather than retrieval ability and reaction time rather than reaction ability are the primary difficulties, perhaps tests emphasizing time factors are not appropriate measurement tools for the elderly. *The clinical implication is that no time pressure must be perceived by the patient, since it is known to distort the patient's ability to participate in and benefit from therapy.* Similarly, a therapist who is impatient and who repeats commands related to a task rather than allowing the elderly client time to process and respond to the first instruction may cause confusion and frustration for patient—and therefore a poor treatment outcome.

Cognitive tasks such as problem-solving ability, spatial–perceptual ability, and word fluency have been reported to change with advanced age.[29,34–36] If one accepts developmental principles regarding the interaction of spatial perception and praxis, and accepts also that both perceptual skills proceed from various additional perceptual functions, one can hypothesize that with aging an individual will have difficulty with (1) planning movement, (2) negotiating space while moving, (3) determining alternative solutions through reasoning, and (4) correcting errors such as loss of balance with adequate speed.

Loss of efficiency of normal input and sensory systems, CNS degeneration, central processing problems, slowness in reaction time, and generalized deterioration of the muscular system will definitely affect the results of any physical or occupational therapy evaluation. If these changes occur in our normal, healthy elderly population, how can a health professional determine whether the evaluation results recorded are of acute or chronic origin?

Implications for Treatment

Although clinicians cannot answer the above question, some suggestions regarding treatment may be of benefit to the reader. *Direct feedback with some delay and without immediate introduction of a new stimulus will create a more optimal condition for learning.*[37] Instruction in visual imagery and, possibly, presentation of a visual stimulus representing an appropriate image may facilitate a client's learning or relearning process, if the client's visual perceptual system is intact.[38] Using intramodality learning sequences,[17] such as asking a client (once a therapist has normalized tone) to align himself to vertical while the therapist applies various proprioceptive input modalities such as approximation and primary stretch, should aid learning. The therapist may also guide a client through a movement sequence using a handling technique before asking the client to motor plan the task. Limiting the degree of extraneous input or interference assists in memory, recall, and learning. Determining differences between sensory acuity and central processing difficulty, as well as the minimal level of functional use of both areas with regard to learning is vital if more adequate treatment techniques are to be developed in order to help our elderly population regain skills needed for ADL.

Role of the Limbic System

The client's emotional needs and attitude toward both therapy and life not only reflect the cognitive-perceptual functioning of the brain, but also the emotional system (limbic) responses. The limbic system directs many aspects of CNS processing. Fear can drastically affect both memory and learning. Fear of falling, of failing, of being rejected, of growing old, and of losing power and status can hamper the optimal effectiveness of a therapy session. The client's attitude is often reflected in willingness to participate in therapy. Even a person who is 85 years of age still has the right to make decisions, to feel important, and to be respected. We, as clinicians, wish to feel important, desire respect, and need to make decisions. Yet imagine being a 24-year-old therapist working with a 93-year-old amputee. The client was 69 years old when the therapist was born. Which person, in the perception of the patient is the wisest, most mature, and most responsible for making decisions? Mutual rather than disproportionate respect will generally lead to a better environment for learning.

Individuality of the Client

The client's previous learning plays a remarkably profound role in the client's treatment. This is true not only in the area of learning styles and interests, but also in the area of emotional and social learning. Through 60 to

100 years of life, the client has developed a perception of the world and a filtering system that allows maintenance of that perception. Two people having the same experience may view it in drastically different ways. One client will perceive the experience as devastating and negative and gain nothing from it but pain, whereas the next client will perceive it as a learning experience. The former will probably see her or his disability in a negative light and the latter will try to adapt to it and grow from it. *It is the therapist's role not to change the client's perceptual world but to accept it and help the client benefit from therapy as best as is possible.*

Closely related to perceptual filters are stereotypes. The client has "learned" how devastating disabilities are and has "learned" how disabled persons act. On becoming disabled, the elderly client may fulfill the role of being disabled by engaging in such stereotyped behaviors. A client who perceives the elderly and disabled as dependent, may become much more dependent (especially if he or she is inclined to be dependent). The elderly are sometimes stereotyped as angry, confused, eccentric, and intolerant of others. All of these stereotypes may be adopted by a client who now has a good excuse to display these behaviors and sees no need to expend the energy to inhibit them any more. Some behaviors may have an organic base, such as spontaneous swearing after a CVA. The therapist must be keenly aware of the client's inner perceptions in order to establish the rapport necessary to build the trusting relationship necessary to promote adequate therapeutic change.

Trust is the Basis for Therapy

Trust is a basic element of a therapeutic relationship. Without trust, the person in need of therapy will find it hard to risk possible damage to his or her physical, emotional, and social being. It is obvious that the client must trust the therapist not to let the client fall or come to physical harm, but the client must also trust the therapist to create an environment that will not allow the client to suffer ego loss due to failure and/or social disgrace due to public humiliation. Without this trust, the client must expend extra energy in protecting himself or herself, thus draining energy and concentration from what is to be learned in therapy and making therapy less efficient. Finally, the client must trust the therapist to create an environment that will promote growth and make the output of the client's time, energy, and money worthwhile. Thus, the gifted therapist must be aware of all aspects of the client's behavioral responses, CNS functioning, and learning environment in order to attain optimal functioning of the client.

Client's External Environment

All stimuli surrounding the patient make up the external environment. People, noises, lighting, furniture, smells, etc., all act as input to the client's inner world. Familiar input such as home, friend, grandma's beef stew, and a familiar alarm clock, rather than the unfamiliar input of hospital, strangers, institutional food, and a wake-up call, help the client match information with previous learning. Thus, maintaining a sensorially rich and *familiar* external environment rather than deprived, strange surroundings should help orient the client and promote optimal growth. Nevertheless, a rich environment does not mean an indiscriminate bombardment of the client's sensory world. Extraneous noise, lighting, or people may confuse or overload a client's processing system, thus decreasing efficiency. The input provided must be adapted to the individual needs of each patient throughout the day.

Therapist's Internal World

The therapist, as a partner in the therapeutic process, has preferential or primary learning styles, adaptive processes, attitudes toward life and people, and ways of dealing with numerous different situations. As a student, the therapist had to learn to adapt to the ways in which teachers wished the therapist to learn in order to perform well on tests. Most of us have had at least one teacher to whom we could never adapt no matter how hard we studied. Thus, we never did well on that teacher's tests although we may have known the material better than the teacher.

The therapist who becomes the teacher or clinician may either fall into the same cycle of expecting students or clients to adapt to the way the therapist teaches most comfortably or may create environments in which clients can optimally learn in their best and easiest learning style. Gifted therapists seem to sense how to create that environment for patients.

The therapist who understand his or her own preferential learning styles and ways to adapt is beginning to understand the multitudinous ways in which the learning environment for clients can and cannot be changed. For example, if the therapists and the client's primary style is visual-spatial, the client should comprehend optimally when the therapist demonstrates a motor task. On the other hand, if the therapist's style is verbal and the client's is visual-spatial, the therapist must make a choice. If the therapist's style is chosen, the movement must be verbally described to your client. If the client's mode is selected, the therapist must demonstrate visually to the client. Obviously, if the therapist verbally describes and the client fails, another method should be tried. Yet, between the time of the first attempt and a second attempt with a better method, the client would have experienced lack of success (failure). This situation tends to decrease motivation, increase frustration, and often creates a gap between the therapist and client.

Clinician's External World

Just as clients have ordinary daily worlds surrounding them, so do therapists. That external world can alter a therapist's internal processing and response patterns. Stress in personal life may carry over into a therapist's work.

For example, if I am upset and wish to be alone but come to work, I will try to isolate myself whenever possible. Assume that Mr. Adams, a 78-year-old man with right CVA comes to the clinic early every day to socialize. Today, instead of inviting him into my office, I tell him to stroll over to the table mat, lock his chair, and wait. I have by my actions told him something is wrong, but not what the problem is. He, being intelligent and observant, will probably assume he did something wrong. This assumption is made because I am the professional and "Nothing bothers me." When I begin to treat Mr. Adams, I will probably note an increase in tone and ask him if something is bothering him. My external world will have altered my internal responses and in turn have altered Mr. Adams' external world, affecting his internal world and creating hypertonicity. The emotional input can make his control over his body more stressful, possibly further increasing the tone and decreasing the effectiveness of the treatment session.

If instead of avoiding sharing my pain, I tell Mr. Adams that I am having a bad day, I will have changed the previous environment totally. Mr. Adams will realize that he is not the problem; this should decrease his anxiety and avoid creating limbic responses and hypertonicity. It also lets the client know it is all right to have bad as well as good days. That is, it is perfectly acceptable to feel bad. I have also created a situation which allows Mr. Adams to ask me if he can help me. He is then the potential provider and I the receiver. This interaction is a goal of all rehabilitation services—independence and interdependence.

Awareness of your actions, what effects them, and how they are received by clients is another key element in creating an optimal learning environment. Getting to know yourself precedes truly getting to know your clients.

CONCLUSION

Life encompasses a series of responses directly related to the demands placed upon us. At each phase of our life, the specific demands and available response patterns vary. The complex characteristics of a healthy person at specific phases of development must first be understood if accurate analysis of that person's potential following illness or acute external or internal insult to the body is to be made. Elderly persons, their experiences, their beliefs, their fears, their available physical and emotional resources, and their problems, play a key role in society's balance. A clinician's sensitivity and awareness of the unique, varied, and normal responses of an older client can help reinforce the positive attributes of that person while dealing with dysfunctions in a more productive way. An understanding of the available behavioral responses and their limitation due to age allows the therapist to break down activities into components and reorganize those needed skills so that the elderly person can feel success. The introduction of normal movement experiences helps reorient the client to both past learning and current demands.

The best method of introducing sensory input, whether it be verbal through words, kinesthetic through handling techniques, or visual through imitation, depends not only on the intact sensory world of the client, but also on the primary receiving, processing, and planning sensory systems that control the behavioral output of the client. The normal functioning of an adult CNS as well as the ongoing changes incurred in the brain and peripheral systems with age also plays an important role in establishing priorities for appropriate therapeutic procedures when an optimal clinical setting for an elderly person that will maximize therapeutic receptiveness is created. One must consider: (1) familiarity with the surrounding environment, (2) consistency with the daily routine, (3) goal setting and treatment sequencing based on appropriate needs, and (4) balancing expectations and abilities, all intertwined.

Not only are the general characteristics of aging important with regard to the normal internal mechanism of the elderly person and the external expectations of society, but the individual features unique to each client must also be evaluated and respected. The client's learning styles, emotional integrity, biorhythms, needs, experiences, and support system, are all factors in the client–therapist clinical learning environment. Each component and many others can alter the moment-to-moment changes surrounding the client and thus alter the response patterns. Yet these changes in behaviors should be seen only as slight alterations in the behavioral responses observed regularly in adults. In a normally changing environment, abrupt behavioral deviations are not normal. Rapid changes in tone (versus slow deterioration of muscle function), acute dementia (versus slow decline in mental abilities), and rapid equilibrium loss (versus slow decrease in balance abilities) are not signs of aging. Aging is an ongoing process of slow change from the moment of conception. Acute change is caused by some accelerated process of illness or trauma that can occur at any age.

A clinician must analyze the response or behaviors of clients according to reality, not mythology. Whether life continues or ends with old age is determined by attitude. All of us have an opportunity to experience the full spectrum of life. Placing oneself both physically and emotionally in the role of the recipient of therapy helps a clinician develop both respect and sensitivity to the needs, frustrations, pain, and joys of the client. Knowing that at sometime the therapist may be in the receiving role makes one ask: "If it were I, how would I wish to be perceived, interacted with, and treated?" If that question remains at the level of sensitivity necessary to create change, the clinician will always be aware of the true needs of the client and allow that unique person to reach his or her desired expectation.

ACKNOWLEDGMENT

We thank Jeb Burton for his artistic contributions.

REFERENCES

1. Umphred D, McCormack GL: Classification of common facilitatory and inhibitory treatment techniques. p. 72. In Umphred D (ed): Neurological Rehabilitation. CV Mosby, St. Louis, 1985
2. Umphred D: An integrated approach to treatment of the pediatric neurologic patient. p. 89. In Campbell SK (ed): Pediatric Neurologic Physical Therapy. Churchill Livingstone, New York, 1984
3. Pickles B: Biological aspects of aging. p. 27. In Jackson O (ed) Physical Therapy of the Geriatric Patient, Churchill Livingstone, New York, 1983
4. Critchley M: Neurology of old age. Lancet 1:1119, 1931
5. Hunziker O, Abdel'Al S, Schulz U: The aging human cerebral cortex: a stereological characterization of changes in the capillary net. J Gerontol 34:345, 1979
6. Libow L: Medical investigation of the process of aging. Ch. 5. In Human Aging: A Biological and Behavioral Study, United States Department of Health, Education and Welfare, Washington, D.C., 1962
7. Heikkinen E, Kiiskinen A, Kayhty B, et al: Assessment of biological age: methodological study in two Finnish populations. Gerontologia 20:33, 1974
8. Dastur DF, Lane MH, Hansen DB, et al: Effects of aging on cerebral circulation and metabolism in man. Ch. 6. In Human Aging: a Biological and Behavioral Study. United States Department of Health, Education and Welfare, Washington, D.C., 1963
9. Frolkis VV: Regulation process in the mechanism of aging. Exp Gerontol 3:113, 1969
10. Corso JF: Sensory processes and age effects in normal adults. J Gerontol 26:90, 1971
11. Botwinich J: Aging and Behavior. Springer, New York, 1973
12. Hurwitz LJ, Swallow M: An introduction to the neurology of aging. Gerontol Clin 13:97, 1971
13. Serratrice G, Roux H, Aquaron R: Proximal muscle weakness in elderly subjects. J Neurol Sci 7:279, 1968
14. Bolton CF, Winkelmann RK, Dyck PJ: A quantitative study of Meissner's corpuscles in man. Neurology 16:1, 1966
15. Sheldon JH: On the natural history of falls in old age. Br Med J 4:1685, 1960
16. Murray MP, Clarkson BH: The vertical pathways of the foot during level walking. J Am Phys Ther Assoc 46:586, 1966
17. Murray MP, Kory RC, Clarkson BH: Walking patterns in healthy old men. J Gerontol 24:169, 1969
18. Finley FR, Cody KA, Finizie, RV: Locomotion patterns in elderly women. Arch Phys Med 50:140, 1969
19. Hass A, Russ HA, Persof H, et al: Respiratory function in hemiplegic patients. Arch Phys Med 48:174, 1967
20. Hellebrandt FA, Houtz SJ, Petridge MJ, et al: Tonic neck reflexes in exercises of stress in man. Am J Phys Med 35:144, 1956
21. Paulson G, Gottlieb G: Developmental reflexes: the reappearance of fetal and neonatal reflexes in aged patients. Brain 91:37, 1968
22. Waterland JC, Hellebrandt FA: Involuntary patterning associated with willed movement performed against progressively increased resistance. Am J Phys Med 43:13, 1964
23. Bobath B: Adult Hemiplegia: Evaluation and Treatment. Heinemann, London, 1970

24. Brunnstrom S: Movement Therapy in Hemiplegia. Harper and Row, New York, 1970

25. Dasco MM, Luczak AK, Rush HA: Bracing and rehabilitation training: effect on energy expenditure of the olderly hemiplegic. Preliminary report. Postgrad Med 34:42, 1963

26. Corcoran J, Jebsen R, Brengelmann G, et al: Effects of plastic and metal leg braces on speed and energy cost of hemiparetic patients. Arch Phys Med Rehab 57:69, 1970

27. Hirschberg GG, Ralson HJ: Energy cost of stair climbing in normal and hemiplegic subjects. Am J Phys Med 44:165, 1965

28. Schaie KW, LaBouvie GV: Generational versus ontogenetic components of change in adult cognitive behavior: a fourteen-year cross-sequential study. Dev Psychol 10:305, 1974

29. Schaie KW, LaBouvie GV, Buech BU: Generational and cohort-specific differences in adult and cognitive functioning. Dev Psychol 9:151, 1973

30. Spirduso WW, Clifford P: Replication of age and physical activity effects on reaction and movement. J Gerontol 33:26, 1978

31. Rotella RJ, Bunker LK: Field dependence and reaction time in senior tennis players (65 and over). Percept Mot Skills 46:585, 1978

32. Kemp BS: Reaction time of young and elderly subjects in relation to perceptual deprivation and signal-on versus signal-off conditions. Dev Psychol 8:268, 1973

33. Anders TR, Fozard JL, Lillyquist TD: Effects of age upon retrieval for short-term memory. Dev Psychol 9:214, 1972

34. Arenberg D: A longitudinal study of problems solving in adults. J Gerontol 29:650, 1974

35. Elias MF: Age and sex differences in relationship in the processing of verbal and nonverbal stimuli. J Gerontol 29:162, 1974

36. Hayslip B, Sterns HL: Age differences in relationship between crystallized and fluid intelligence and problem solving. J Gerontol 34:404, 1979

37. Ward LC, Maisto AA: The effects of delay, type and duration of feedback on verbal-discrimination learning. Am J Psychol 86:547, 1973

38. Groninger LD: The role of images within the memory system—storage or retrieval? J Exp Psychol 130:178, 1974

4 | Breathing: An Approach for Facilitating Movement

Carola H. Speads
Margaret J. Leong

My (CHS) approach of working with breathing derives from my studies with Elsa Gindler (1885–1961). She was the most advanced of the teachers in the field of body work in Germany. I studied with her for many years and taught with her and for her. Her approach, consisting of not exercise but of trying to have students feel their bodily condition and to experiment and find ways to improve it was unique then.[1-5]

The support of breathing is as important for the physical therapist and the occupational therapist as it is for their patients. Therapists often must lift, support, or shift the weight of patients, stand for extended periods, and walk the long hallways of a hospital or nursing home. The elderly need the support of their breathing to move impaired limbs or their stiffer or weaker bodies. Patients may have to reacquire former skills or learn new ways to achieve them again. Pain and anxiety often overshadow such strivings and thus interfere with breathing,[6-8] or these difficulties are actually created and sustained by poor breathing. In fact, poor breathing may even make it impossible to overcome handicaps; it curtails endurance, causes dizziness, and creates and sustains feelings of insecurity[9] and thus anxieties, such as the fear of falling[10,11] or of dropping things. The support through facilitation of breathing, however, will ease such tasks, help to overcome handicaps, and thus make the rehabilitation program more effective.

Experience with becoming aware of breathing conditions and of monitoring the facilitation process of breathing, however, is imperative, and must be acquired. This means, primarily, that the quality of the patient's breathing should not be left to chance but must be recognized by both therapist and patient. Therapists should be able to observe clearly their patient's ways of breathing at rest as well as when they are moving around or with becoming aware of breathing conditions and of performing the activities of daily living (ADL). They can do this only after having gathered experience with their own ways of breathing, that is, once they have learned to recognize the ways in which their breathing can respond to facilitation and enhance or obstruct their own performance of ADL.

GUIDELINES FOR RECOGNIZING AND EVALUATING QUALITY OF BREATHING

Some patients easily verbalize what they feel about how their breathing is working and how they respond to attempts to improve it. Other patients may not be so communicative, and some patients may not be able to speak about it at all. Therapists, therefore, should be trained to observe and to recognize the signs of how effectively a patient's breathing is working so they do not have to rely solely on monitoring blood pressure, pulse rate, and respiratory cycles per minute.

Close observation of many patients will develop into a skill, so that eventually the main features of a patient's breathing will almost instantly be recognized by the therapist. Continued observation of the same patient will, of course, give more detailed insight. Some hints of what to look for and how to assess the quality of a patient's breathing follow.

Posture

Some disturbances of breathing, of course, are quite obvious, easily observed, like fighting for breath, heaving, or making involuntary noises with inhalation or exhalation. The posture of the patient is also a key to breathing quality. It should be observed when the patient is lying, sitting, and moving. Is the thorax squeezed together? Are the shoulders pulled up, held tightly squeezed toward the neck, or are they hanging flabbily forward? What is the general muscle tone: hypertense or hypotense? Tonus influences the quality of breathing; observing it therefore gives a hint as to how to begin to facilitate an easy and effective ventilation.

How is the patient lying? Patients should lie in the position most comfortable for them. The therapist should observe whether the patient is really resting comfortably or attempting to maintain the body off the surface on which it is lying. Is the patient in the opposite state, a state of collapse?

How is the patient sitting? Is the patient balancing on the tuber ischiadicum so that the trunk is upright, or too far back on it, therefore having to bend the upper thorax forward? A forward bending would cause squeezing together of the front of the thorax, resulting in an overcontraction of the chest cage and diaphragm and pressure on the abdominal content, which would be visible by its protrusion. In the opposite manner of sitting, the patient sits too far forward on the tuber ischiadicum, showing a hollow in the small of the back and a protruding abdomen, thus causing poor breathing in the area of the lower back. In both sitting positions described, it is impossible for the diaphragm to work freely and, as a result, breathing is less effective.

Hollows above and below the clavicles can be seen easily and indicate poor breathing in these areas—the tips of the lungs. Watch for the *rhythm of breathing* as well. Is it regular, irregular, too fast or too slow?

Observe the movement of the whole thorax. How much movement is there? If there is too much movement, an extra effort is noticeable in breathing. If there is almost no thoracic movement, sluggish breathing resulting in insufficient oxygen will be noted.

Does the patient *sigh* from time to time? Sighing indicates poor breathing quality and forced, deeper exhalations. It is a forced exhalation and thus a means to produce deeper inhalations.

Observe whether the patient tends to *stop* breathing every so often or holds his breath when striving to achieve a task. Obviously, this would deprive the patient of the support of his breathing. It should be mentioned that only for lifting or pushing heavy objects is a holding of the breath necessary to give the arms a firm base on the thorax from which to work.

Note: It is usually unimportant whether a movement is started on inhalation or finished on exhalation. An elderly or handicapped person in particular may need more time to execute a movement than one phase of breathing can provide. *The key thing is that breathing must not be interfered with*, that the patient does not obstruct his breathing.[12,13] Only if the breathing flows freely will the patient have an adequate supply of energy available. This, in turn, means less strain, more endurance, less anxiety, more confidence, and last but not least, a better mood! As a consequence, the patient will have more courage to tackle the often difficult and physically demanding tasks of rehabilitation.

THEORY AND PRACTICE OF BREATHING WORK

Before discussing the details of breathing work (BRW), I wish to emphasize again that therapists themselves should do BRW. Only when they have experienced what their own breathing feels like, how it reacts to stimuli, and how a better quality of breathing can facilitate movement, will they become able to observe, evaluate, and help to improve the quality of their patients' breathing. Facilitating the quality, quantity, and ease of breathing is relevant whether the patient is at rest, moving, or trying to recover movements impaired by the ordinary afflictions of old age, by injury or disease, or just by a more sedentary life, which often results in a loss of agility.

Experimenting

It is imperative that therapist and patient never forget that breathing is an involuntary function.[13–16] We cannot *make* it. We can only stimulate, *coax, or facilitate it*. We can provide a stimulus and then accommodate the reactions to that stimulus.

Working with stimuli for facilitation, however, is different from working with the concept of exercises. Whereas the success of exercising is based on a more or less mechanical repetition of the same procedure, giving a stimulus and then accommodating the body's reactions to it means *experimenting*—a much more far-reaching and rewarding way of working. Of course, the more the patient is able to let these reactions through, the more far-reaching is the effect of an experiment. Experimenting generally achieves more and gets faster results, and it remains forever interesting. As we are rarely in the same condition, variations of reactions are bound to occur: some superficial, others far-reaching. With experimentation, patients will be less likely to become bored long before their aims are reached, as they often do with exercise. Patients will continue to work with their breathing, as well as with other rehabilitation tasks, as they become increasingly interested in trying movements with the support of their breathing. Furthermore, the power of concentration developed through sustained experimenting is most useful, particularly for the elderly whose power of concentration so often tends to fade (for many reasons).

It is taken for granted that a trained therapist's work will be done gently and with consideration of the overall condition of the patient, so that undue strain, which would inhibit breathing, will be avoided. Of course, BRW with the elderly should at first be done for short periods only. Patients who have not used their breathing properly tend to hyperventilate; only gradually can the body tolerate a larger supply of oxygen. Watch for dizziness, malaise, and overwhelming and sudden tiredness, the signs of hyperventilation. If hyperventilation occurs, the BRW must be interrupted.[16–18] In this case, somewhat vigorous movements, like tapping, swinging the arms, making fists on the chest and throwing the arms out a couple of times will be enough to overcome the hyperventilation. With patients in a hospital or institution, BRW can be tried again after a few hours. If, however, hyperventilation occurs again immediately or shortly thereafter, BRW must be postponed until the following day. This should be explained to patients so that they follow the same procedure when they work alone. Generally speaking, patients should feel better, that is, refreshed, after having done BRW.

Checkup

Most people are aware of their breathing only when it is disturbed, that is, when they feel out of breath. They are unfamiliar with the ordinary quality of their breathing. The first step, therefore, to enable patients to use their breathing to advantage in rehabilitation work is to establish in them a conscious awareness of their breathing. Before starting and after stopping rehabilitation work, time should be taken so that both therapist and patient become aware of the condition of the patient's breathing. Is it sufficient or insufficient to support them during their activities? Most often, BRW will be found necessary. The results of BRW, the improved quality of the breathing that will be achieved, can be fully appreciated and judged correctly only if these two conditions can be compared: (1) Patients should *feel* how they breathe, and (2) therapists should *observe* it.[19,20]

It should be emphasized that we feel neither the healthy lungs nor the diaphragm themselves, but processes related to breathing, such as rib cage expansion, laboring for breath, holding of the breath, breathing only in limited areas, breathing in spurts, breathing with ease, or breathing fluently.

The therapist and patient should also become aware of the breathing condition before attempting to improve because achievement of a more normal breathing condition often is not registered as change or improvement. After all, normal simply feels normal. Only if differences and achievements can be consciously registered is there incentive to pursue efforts for a sustained change in breathing. *A checkup (CHU), therefore, should be done before beginning and when ending a work period.*

The CHU is started by asking patients two questions: Can they feel anything at all in their body that seems to be related to their breathing, and where do they feel it? Everyone, even people rather unrelated to their bodies, will respond to this question. They will describe specific areas as involved, such as the upper chest, abdomen, or nose.

The second question will often be answered before it has been asked: namely, how the breathing works: what its quality is, in what manner it occurs, how it truly feels—labored, easy, fluent, or interrupted. Some people may respond by saying that they cannot answer because they do not feel anything. But often these people later describe clearly and in detail how they feel their breathing to be different from the way it was when they began. That can be interpreted as, they felt it before but not yet consciously.

Someone once described this dilemma: "I feel it, but for the life of me I could not put it into words." Eventually, however, every patient will answer precisely. Therapists should not be surprised if some patients describe impressions of their breathing as color: for example, "It was dark, now it is lighter". They may describe it as weight: "It was heavy, now it has eased up."

To help patients feel changes in the condition of their breathing more easily, it is advisable to work first—if the experiment permits—with one-half of the thorax only. If another CHU is then done at the end of the work period, the differences in the condition between the halves can more easily be felt. The more patients become aware of the good results of their work, the more they will be motivated to work on their own and not only when they are supervised.

Position

Stimuli to breathing can be given with the patient in any body position— lying, sitting, or moving. Use the position that is most comfortable for the patient. If the patient is sitting, the height of the seat (of the chair or the bed) should be such that the thighs are supported horizontally, the feet rest on the floor, and the ankles are positioned vertically below the knees. The back and pelvis may be supported vertically, or, a patient who is able to do so, may sit more forward on the seat so that pelvis and trunk can balance vertically.

Letting Reactions Through

It cannot be emphasized too strongly that when working with stimuli facilitation, both patient and therapist must take whatever time may be necessary to let the reactions to a stimulus through. These reactions may set in with the next breath; for example, the patient may have an involuntary, deeper inhalation or may yawn, a desire to stretch may make itself felt. Reactions may get through only after the same stimulus has been applied repeatedly. Regardless of the time needed, reactions will always get through eventually. If, however, a new stimulus is given while the breathing is still in the process of changing, it will have a negative effect, that is, disturb the breathing.

Breathing Stimuli

Limited space here prevents me (CHS) from giving all the particulars of how to work with breathing stimuli. The book *Ways to Better Breathing* contains a detailed description of how to proceed.[21]

Stimuli that can be used to improve breathing are many and varied. There are stimuli that can be given by the therapist whenever the patient is incapacitated and others that must be done by the patient himself.

Light tapping of the thorax. This stimulus is performed with one hand above and then below the clavicles, and on lateral and dorsal thorax. It can be done by the patient alone or by the therapist. Tapping gently, the tapping hand should feel the shape of the body and adjust to it. No tapping ever, of course, is done on the breast itself. Tapping of the lower front ribs should be done only when the breathing is strong, or it will irritate the breathing.

Giving an extra wide exit for the exhalation. The patient opens the mouth wide during an exhalation, tongue resting on the bottom of the mouth.[21]

Giving a small exit for the exhalation. The patient lets an exhalation pass through a drinking straw or through the barely opened mouth. The special way of exhaling in both these experiments should be repeated only after the breathing has returned to a regular rhythm.[21]

Light pressure with exhalation along the sternum. Pressure is applied on exhalation with one or two fingertips, beginning at the upper end. (Be sure that the patient does not press into the neck.)[21]

Light pressure on exhalation along the costae. Pressure is applied with one or two fingertips along the frontal, lateral, and dorsal costae.[21]

Light pressure into the intercoastal spaces. Pressure is applied as above.[21]

Lifting skinfolds off the thorax. A skinfold is grasped, lifted and released with the following inhalation. Beginning at the lower rim of the thorax, the therapist eventually works along lateral and dorsal costae. The skinfold should be grasped and released gently.[21]

Touch

If a patient can tolerate neither tapping nor pressure on the thorax, touch can be used as a stimulus. Either therapist or patient should put the fingertips of one or two fingers on the thorax, working along or between the costae, on one area at a time, eventually covering the whole thorax. The patient should try to feel where the fingers touch and whether there is a response in the area underneath the finger, trying to facilitate all reactions as much as possible. This results not only in improvement of the breathing but makes patient and therapist keenly aware of the areas in which the breathing does not respond enough and in which it needs improvement. Thus, it is helpful also in planning adequate BRW for rehabilitation.[21]

Exhalation with sounds

The patient hums on m (mmmmm) or exhales on ha (as in palm), or on a sibilant s, or f. The patient exhales on vowels: a (as in palm); e (as in name); i (as in inter); o (as in over); u (as in pool). Consonants can later be combined with various vowels.[21]

Change of Position

A change of position, even the slightest one, is stimulating to breathing. The patient bends the trunk, at first slightly and later more fully, and remains in this position for a while so that the breathing reacts and fuller breaths into the extended half of the thorax can come through. Bending in any direction can be used; for example, the sitting patient can lean the trunk slightly laterally, with support of the hand or forearm if necessary.[21]

Movements

At first, movements should be extremely small and slow. Movements that are easiest for the patient should be used at first. Later, movements that have to be "rehabilitated" should be attempted. Patients should be aware of their breathing before, when starting, during, and after the movement. The therapist should be sure to wait after the movement to let breathing reactions develop freely. A new movement should *be started only after breathing has become even and consistent.* Raising a shoulder or a knee slightly and letting it settle down again are often good movements to begin with. Eventually, movements that are difficult for the patient can be tried.

The patient should become aware of the relationship between movement and breathing whether a limb is involved or the whole body is in action—as in bending, walking, and the myriad ADL. Experiencing movement supported by breathing and recognizing that a strenuous movement can be recuperated from faster through this support will encourage the patient. This, in turn, will make it easier for the geriatric patient to persevere with rehabilitation work.[21]

SPECIFIC EFFECTS OF BREATHING WORK ON REHABILITATION OF GERIATRIC PATIENTS

Aside from the unquestionable advantage of the improvement of breathing, which facilitates any kind of rehabilitation work, specific effects of BRW are particularly helpful for work with a geriatric patient.

Unilateral Response

The effects of breathing facilitation can be felt even beyond the quality of the breathing itself. The condition of the whole body undergoes change. Patients will experience this most easily by doing BRW so as to influence one-half of the thorax. A CHU will then give a clear impression of a particular effect, the unilateral response of the body. Not only will the breathing in this half of the thorax be easier or fuller, but the whole half of the body will be different from the other in a way clearly observable to patient and therapist. Potential benefits are numerous. Muscle tonus will have regulated itself, and will be higher or lower according to need. Joints will be more elastic. Circulation will be stimulated, and the whole half of the body may feel warmer than the other half. Standing up from work performed while sitting, a patient will not only feel the leg of this side to be longer and more alive, but will stand better on this particular leg. It will anchor the patient more firmly on the floor. That the leg can also be moved more easily can be proven by having the patient take a few, slow steps or merely lift each knee slowly a few times. The feeling of secure anchorage on the ground is of importance: For example, in gait training. In addition, the fear of falling, which can be such an obstacle in the course of the therapy, is diminished. Patients will be confident enough to work on walking if they feel more secure on the floor and more mobile in their joints.

Avoiding Dizziness

The quality of breathing is also important in avoiding the problem of dizziness. Elderly persons are often afraid of becoming or actually become dizzy (for example, when they bend over to pick something up from the floor or have to turn around). Most persons habitually hold their breath during such activities and therefore tend to become dizzy. If such patients make a sound with every exhalation, just loud enough so that they themselves can hear it, they will find that they do not become dizzy. Any kind of sound will do; sounding an f or s will do the trick. Patients can easily keep track of their breathing by hearing or missing the sound. As long as they do not stop breathing but let their breathing flow freely, they will not become dizzy when performing most movements associated with ADL.

Facial Expression

Improved breathing also affects facial expression. Elderly patients who may be in pain and have difficulties with movements often have a pained, harsh, facial expression or one that is sad or bewildered. Without mentioning it beforehand, the therapist should ask the patient to look in a mirror after a session of BRW. It is likely that patients will recognize that they look different, less grim, less worn out, better and younger than they ordinarily do. They will then be less resistant to further rehabilitation work.

Effect on Senses

All senses work better when breathing is eased. The patient's vision, touch, and hearing may be greatly improved.

Attention Span

Attention span is also dependent on the quality of breathing. It will increase with improved breathing, thus enabling the geriatric patient to work for longer periods and to follow instructions with greater ease.

Lessening of Discomfort and Pain

Support of breathing will often eliminate minor discomforts and raise the pain threshold. Movements previously out of reach because of pain may become accessible when the patient can use breathing as a support rather than as a way to defy movement.

Endurance

If discomfort and pain diminish, a patient's endurance for rehabilitation work increases. Longer periods of work can be tolerated, and more difficult and demanding tasks can be undertaken. The experience that breathing can support rehabilitation work and that unavoidable strain can be overcome more easily by improving breathing encourages patients to pursue rehabilitation work when the therapist is with them as well as when they work on their own.

Influence on Sleeping

Many geriatric patients are plagued by difficulty in falling asleep or by sleeping in a way that does not refresh them sufficiently, so that they are too tired to work successfully at their rehabilitation. Once patients have some experience with BRW, they can ease their breathing before trying to fall asleep. Lying in their favorite position or in the one they are compelled to lie in, they can exhale consciously several times. They should not "study" this process. They should just *let* the air flow out in the way that is easiest for them, either opening the mouth or humming, perhaps. They will find not only that they fall asleep soon, but also that they awake more refreshed in the morning. They then will do better rehabilitation work, being less tired and less grouchy when the day begins.

Organ Functions

All organs depend in their functioning on the quality of breathing. Breathing can have a particularly impressive influence on bowel movement. Constipation which plagues so many geriatric patients, often disappears rather suddenly as the action of the diaphragm increases as the breathing improves.

SUMMARY

All bodily functions depend on breathing. BRW, therefore, can change not only the quality of breathing but the total functioning of the body, thus facilitating all rehabilitation work. BRW can be done anywhere; no special place, position, clothing, or particular time of day or length of worktime is required. BRW can be done without other people noticing that it is being done. With experience, even short periods of work can bring positive results. A single, freer breath may change the breathing pattern and change the performance and mood of the geriatric patient from anxiety to fortitude, from despair to an acceptance of limitations.

Therapists will become less fatigued when working with the support of their breathing. They will recuperate faster from the unavoidable strain of a workday, be able to use a short period of time to prepare, and become inventive in coping with the challenge in which the next patient will involve them. They will no longer be confined to routine efforts. Rather, new ways of achieving specific aims will occur to them with ease. Most important, however, they will have a new dimension at their disposal for assessing the condition and the progress of their patients.

A better quality of breathing and the experience of the support of breathing for rehabilitation work are vital for the geriatric patients in their work to master certain tasks: getting up from lying or sitting; standing for longer periods; walking, going up and down stairs; fast turns in any direction; carrying weight (ie, grocery bag), overcoming anxiety of falling or of letting things drop; bending over; completing daily activities; remembering; and overcoming either lethargy or overactivity. Support of breathing, which diminishes discomfort, will enable them to work for longer periods at these tasks. Success will brighten their mood, and annoyance and depression will give way to a more positive outlook on life.

In conclusion, I (CHS) want to share with therapists embarking on BRW with geriatric patients the enormous reward and constant discovery that I, in a lifetime in the field, have enjoyed. Sustained BRW is sure to produce beneficial results in the geriatric patient, no matter how infirm the patient may be. This is, I can assure you, endlessly gratifying to therapist and patient alike.

USE OF BREATHING WORK IN REHABILITATION—A CASE STUDY

C. D., an 80-year-old woman, sustained a right cerebrovascular accident and, after 1 month of hospitalization including rehabilitative therapies, was discharged to her home. A physical therapy home-care program was initiated. C. D.'s major limitation was the need for a moderate degree of physical assistance to sit up, stand, and walk with a walker.

Breathing assessment revealed poor quality of breath support. The general factors were frequent occurrences of dizziness and breath-holding when performing ADL. Her rhythm of breathing was too fast after ambulating 15 feet, which was her maximum endurance; a shortness of breath ensued for at least 5 minutes.

Her posture in sitting was too far back on tuber ischiadicum, a 50° angle of posterior pelvic tilt from neutral, with a moderate degree of upper trunk functional kyphosis and a forward head position. The shoulders were pulled upward excessively, especially on the left, and C. D. felt that her head was heavy. Her muscle control on the right side was diminished, and she expressed a fear of falling when upright.

Along with neuromuscular facilitation and training in ADL, a major part of the program involved breathing work. C. D. learned to coordinate breathing by making a sound with each exhalation, and dizziness decreased. As a consequence, C. D. began to gain ease of movement and increased endurance for repetitions of ADL. Simultaneously, an occupational therapy program was carried out, with emphasis on restoration of function in bathing, dressing, and fine motor activities.

Carriage improved as C. D. was taught to sit vertically on tuber ischiadicum, resulting in a decrease in the degree of functional thoracic kyphosis and forward head posture. Trunk and breath control increased, primarily through breathing work to change the position (lateral trunk lean while resting on forearms) of her elbows, with extra-wide exit exhalations and lifting of skinfolds off the thorax. C. D. developed greater muscle control and less excessive holding of shoulders upward by being taught extremely small, slow movements coordinated with breathing.

C. D. carried out a home program of exercise, assisted by her devoted husband, and developed skill in kinesthetic sensing through the CHU before and after applying breathing stimuli. Her pleasure in noticing motor, breath, and ADL improvement increased her motivation and helped her overcome the depression over her disabilities.

She developed an effective feedback system, knowing when to stop walking and rest when she sensed diminished breath support outdoors. This involved a BRW experiment (usually light pressure with exhalation along the sternum) for rejuvenation so that walking could be resumed.

Her recuperation brought her to independent bed mobility; independent ambulation with a quad cane indoors; ambulation, with the cane and supervised, outdoors for a distance of up to 250 yards; and ascending and descending a flight of stairs and a bus step with infrequent dizziness and no shortness of breath.

At discharge for home PT, C. D. was given a written home program, primarily focusing on BRW, which she learned to carry out independently. She wanted to continue the recuperative process of building endurance to reach her final goal of enjoying a vacation at a mountain resort.

REFERENCES

1. Gindler E: Die Gymnastik des Berufsmenschens 1926 in Gymnastik, Zeitschrift des deutschen Gymnastikbundes, Berlin
2. Stolze H: Die Konzentrative Bewegungstherapie. Mensch und Leben, Verlags and Vertriebs G mb H, Berlin, 1984
3. Hilker F: Elsa Gindler, in Bildung und Erziehung. 14 Jahrg. No. 2. February 1961
4. Speads CH: Elsa Gindler. Aufbau, an American Weekly, Vol. XXVII No. 5
5. Wilhelm R: Elsa Gindler, in Heilkunde-Heilwege 1961, 11 Jahrg. No. 5
6. Darwin C: The Expression of Emotion in Man and Animals. Murray, London, 1872
7. Cannon WB: Bodily Changes in Pain Hunger, Fear and Rage. Norton, New York, 1939
8. Dudley D: Psychophysiology of Respiration in Health and Disease. Appleton-Century-Crofts, New York 1969
9. Selye H: The Stress of Life, McGraw-Hill, New York, 1956
10. Feldenkrais M: Body and Mature Behavior, A Study of Anxiety, Gravitation and Learning. International Universities Press, New York, 1979
11. Bhala R, O'Donnell J, Thoppil E: Ptophobia, phobic fear of falling and its clinical management, Phys Tehrapy 62:2, 1982
12. Krauss H: Atemtherapie, 2nd Ed. Hippoktates Verlag, Stuttgart, 1984
13. Heyer-Grote L: Atemschulung als Element der Psychotherapie. Wissenschaftliche Buchgesellschaft, Darmstadt, 1970

14. Cherniack RM, Cherniack L: Respiration in Health and Disease. WB Saunders, Philadelphia, 1961
15. Bouhuys A: The Physiology of Breathing. Grune & Stratton, Orlando, Fla, 1977
16. Taber W: Taber's Cyclopedic Medical Dictionary. FA Davis, Philadelphia, 1981
17. Shepard RS: Human Physiology. JB Lippincott, Philadelphia, 1971
18. Kofler Leo: The Art of Breathing as the Basis of Tone Production. New York, 1889 in German 23rd Ed. Baerenreiter Verlag, Cassel, 1966
19. Schlafstoerungen C, Andersen H: Atmung u. Stimme, Moeseler Verlag, Wolfenbuettel, 1955
20. Schaarschuch A: Loesungs-und Atemtherapie bei Schlafstoesrungen, Turm Verlag, Bietigheim, 1962
21. Speads CH: Ways to Better Breathing. 2nd ed. Felix Morrow, Great Neck, NY, 1986

5 | Thermoregulation and Use of Heat and Cold

Tim Kauffman

Physical modalities of heat and cold are commonly used to treat pain and dysfunction in patients of all ages. However, with increasing age, attenuation in the physiology, especially in the integument, circulation, and nervous system, may seriously decrease the body's response to ambient or locally applied temperature gradients. These changes must be considered when thermal effects are desired in the care and treatment of elderly persons, especially those who are past the seventh decade of life.

The therapeutic consideration to use heat or cold with elderly persons is particularly important because aging is characterized by chronic pathological processes such as heart disease, arthritis, circulatory impairment, and complications such as pain and bed-rest deconditioning. These conditions result from the age-related declining ability to maintain and repair body cells, tissues, and organs.[1,2] This progressive diminution affects body systems and homeostasis, including thermoregulation.[3] These systemic or holistic considerations are important because the body's core temperature and the mechanism for its homeostasis are not inseparable from the local tissue effects resulting from the application of heat and cold.

BASIC CONCEPTS AND LAWS OF THERMODYNAMICS

Before we proceed to therapeutic considerations, some of the basic concepts of heat and thermal dynamics must be briefly stated. First, *thermal energy* is the total kinetic energy of molecular motion in a system. *Heat* is a particular form of energy exchange or transfer between two systems because of temperature differences. *Cold* is the relative absence of heat. *Temperature* is an arbitrary scale with defined units of degrees assigned to a level of internal energy.

The *Zeroith Law* of thermal dynamics indicates that if body A is in statistical equilibrium with body B, and body B is in statistical equilibrium with body C, then C is in statistical equilibrium with A and if C is placed in contact with A, there is no transfer of energy between them. The *first law of thermal dynamics* states that the heat added to a system is equal to the increase in the internal energy of the system plus the work done by the system against its surroundings. The *second law of thermal dynamics* states that when a system containing a large number of particles is left to itself, it assumes a state with maximal entropy; that is, it becomes as disordered as possible. The *third law of thermal dynamics* states that a system in equilibrium at the absolute zero of temperature is in a state of perfect order and has zero entropy.

The clinical significance is that heat will be transferred from the area of greater temperature to the area of lesser temperature. For instance, when a hydrocollator pack of 77°C is applied to skin with a temperature of ~32°C, the heat energy will be transferred from the pack to the skin. On the contrary, when a cold pack with a temperature of ~7°C is applied, the heat will transfer from the skin to the pack, thereby lowering the skin temperature. The flow of heat is an attempt to equalize the temperature between the surfaces; however, it is much more complex because the body will respond to the temperature change to prevent tissue damage. (See Appendix 5-1 for a conversion of Centigrade to Fahrenheit scales.)

HEAT TRANSFER

Several methods of heat (cold) transfer concern us. First, in the example above in which a hydrocollator pack is applied to skin, heat will move from the warmer to the cooler object by the process of conduction. The vascular response to this is vasodilatation, and the blood is heated. The heated blood (or cooled blood in the case of cryotherapy) transfers the heat to adjacent body areas by the process of convection. Transfer of heat by forced convection takes place outside the body by the movement of air or water coming in contact with the skin.

Radiation is another method of heat transfer that greatly influences body temperature and consequently the effects of therapeutically applied heat or cold. When the temperature of an object (in this case, the human body) is above absolute zero, electromagnetic waves are emitted from the "hot body." The human body emits thermal radiation predominantly in the infrared wavelength of the electromagnetic spectrum.[4] At normal room temperature, ~60 percent of total heat loss from a nude body occurs by this radiation method of heat transfer.[5]

Evaporation is another mechanism of heat transport from the body. An uncontrollable amount of water evaporates insensibly by diffusing through the skin and by exhaling air from the lungs. For each gram of water that evaporates,

0.58 calories of heat are lost.[5] Sweating, an additional active evaporative process, involves the eccrine glands that are regulated by the autonomic nervous system. Humidity has a predominant influence on this method of heat transport: the less humidity, the more heat loss can occur by evaporation.

These methods of heat transfer are important for clinicians to consider when applying heat and cold therapeutically. What tissues are conducting the heat? What insulation does the aged integument offer to convection? Is the evaporation process the same in the 25-year-old patient as in the 85-year-old patient? The ambient temperature, humidity, patient's clothing, air currents, treatment surface, and mode of application will affect the transfer of heat.

REGULATION OF BODY TEMPERATURE

All the above concepts and mechanisms are involved in the isothermal system of the normal adult who maintains a core body temperature of 36 to 38°C. Rectal temperatures are generally ~.56°C higher than oral temperatures, and measurements taken earlier in the morning are generally .56°C cooler than those taken later in the day.[5]

Skin temperature varies from core temperature and from one skin location to another. The skin temperatures of the head, face, and trunk are generally closer to core temperature than are the skin temperatures of the hands and feet.[6] The range of skin temperature appears to widen with increasing age (Fig. 5-1).

Body heat which results largely from metabolism is regulated by cardiovascular, hormonal, and nervous control. The temperature-regulating center, or thermostat, is located in the hypothalamus. The heat-sensitive neurons of the preoptic area of the hypothalamus are thought to be the most important. Heat and cold sensory receptors in the skin also transmit impulses to the spinal cord and thus to the hypothalamic control center.[7] Other temperature receptors are found in the spinal cord, abdomen, and muscles.[8] These signals are received in the posterior hypothalamus and are integrated with impulses from the preoptic area.

Nonthermal efffects also play a role in the sophisticated process of thermoregulation, especially during exercise. These factors include: increase in arterial pressure, firing of joint and muscle mechanoreceptors, impulses from the chemosensitive nerve endings in the exercising muscle, changes in central blood volume and plasma electrolytes, depletion of glycogen, and pooling of blood in the periphery.[9]

RESPONSE TO HEAT

Through complex homeostatic mechanisms, the hypothalamic thermostat maintains the body core temperature. If the core temperature goes above 37.3°C the preoptic area of the hypothalamus inhibits the normal sympathetic control

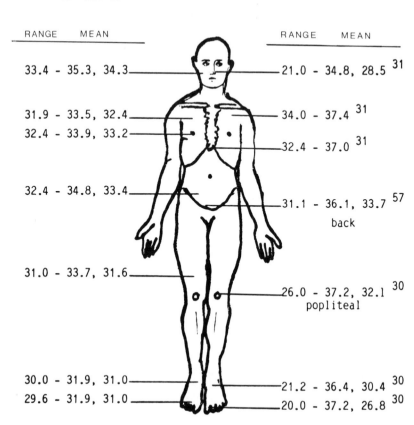

Young
Dermatomes

Old

RANGE	MEAN		RANGE	MEAN

33.4 - 35.3, 34.3 ———— 21.0 - 34.8, 28.5 [31]

31.9 - 33.5, 32.4 ———— 34.0 - 37.4 [31]
32.4 - 33.9, 33.2 ———— 32.4 - 37.0 [31]

32.4 - 34.8, 33.4 ———— 31.1 - 36.1, 33.7 [57]
back

31.0 - 33.7, 31.6 ———— 26.0 - 37.2, 32.1 [30]
popliteal

30.0 - 31.9, 31.0 ———— 21.2 - 36.4, 30.4 [30]
29.6 - 31.9, 31.0 ———— 20.0 - 37.2, 26.8 [30]

Fig. 5-1. A sample of skin temperature of young and old adults. Measurements of skin temperature were made by various investigators with different instruments under resting conditions without extreme ambient temperatures or humidity. When possible, range and mean Centigrade temperatures are reported. Superscript numbers refer to references.

of vasoconstriction. The resultant change in vasomotor tone allows vasodilatation of the skin blood vessels and consequential heat loss by conduction and convection.

Concomitantly, when the preoptic area of the hypothalamus is heated, active sweating is stimulated, allowing heat loss through evaporation. In addition to the hypothalamus thermostat, sweating may be stimulated by heating of certain centers in the spinal cord which evokes the sympathetic response of reduced vasoconstriction. Increased sweat gland activity may also directly increase vasodilatation, which further enhances heat loss.[5] Local skin temperature has an important modifying influence on sweating rate.[10,11]

It is only the eccrine sweat glands, of which there are 2 to 3 million covering the entire body, that are involved in heat loss. The apocrine glands are found in association with pilosebaceous structures, particularly in the axillae, anogenital, and mammary regions of the body. The milky fluid released from the apocrine glands is not related to heat loss.

RESPONSE TO COLD

When the core temperature is lowered from 37.3°C, the body response is to conserve the heat that it has and, if necessary, to produce more heat. Cooling of the body stimulates sympathetic nerve centers that cause vasoconstriction and stop sweating. Piloerection also results from cold stimulation of the hypothalamus. The skin, and especially the subcutaneous fat, insulate the core body temperature from the ambient temperature. Fat does not conduct heat as well as other tissues do. With vasoconstriction, the body is less able to radiate and conduct heat to the environment.

Despite sympathetic vasoconstriction, the body may have to increase its heat production. This is partially achieved by excitation of the primary motor center for shivering located in the posterior hypothalamus. Impulses from cold sensors in the skin and spinal cord stimulate the posterior hypothalamus, which consequently increases skeletal muscle tone. Shivering begins if the skeletal muscle tone reaches a threshold level for the muscle spindle stretch reflex.[5]

Cellular metabolism may also be increased by sympathetic stimulation and by changes in blood levels of norepinephrine and epinephrine. Adrenal and thyroid influences may also contribute to heat production by increasing cell metabolism. These latter two mechanisms are thought to be involved after a person has been exposed to cold for several weeks.[5]

Perceptions involving psychological processes are also involved in thermal regulation. When the hypothalamic thermostat is heated, a psychic response of feeling too warm causes a person to take appropriate action. Likewise, cooling of the thermostat and/or cooling of the skin receptors elicits a perception of feeling too cold. In response, one curls up into a ball, puts on more clothing, or may even start jumping, stamping, or rubbing.[12] What determines physical comfort/discomfort involves interactions between psychological processes and physiological controls that have just been described.[13]

PERIPHERAL SKIN THERMORECEPTORS

Thus far, the sensory receptors for thermal stimuli have been mentioned only briefly; the focus has been on the central receptors, specifically in the spinal cord and the hypothalamus. The understanding of skin thermoreceptors is unclear. Morphologically, it was thought that the heat receptors were Ruffini's end organs, and cold receptors were Krause's end bulbs.[12] Anatomically, these structures cannot be denied, but physiologically this delineation has not been clarified.[14-16] It is now accepted that peripheral thermoreceptors are free

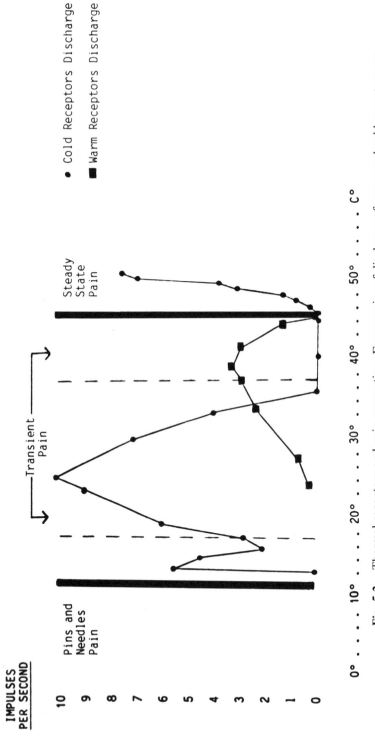

Fig. 5-2. Thermal receptors and pain perception. Frequencies of discharge of warm and cold receptors are from Zotterman.[15] The pain receptors are spurious thermoreceptors as described by Hensel.[14] Cold pain perception data are from Wolfe and Hardy.[52] Heat pain perception data are from Neisser[18] and Hardy and Stolwijk.[58]

nerve endings with terminals passing into the basal epidermal cells of the integument.[14] What causes the depolarization of these nerve endings has not been elucidated; however, thermal perception involves interpretations of the impulses from cold, warm, pain, and possibly mechanical receptors (Fig. 5-2).[5,14-18]

Pain nerve endings fire at extreme warm or cold temperatures, at ~45 and ~15°C, respectively.[17] Cold receptors discharge from ~5 to 43°C[14] and again at 45°C.[15] Warm receptors discharge in the temperature range of 25 to 45°C. Maximal frequency of discharge is in the 25 to 35°C range for cold receptors and in the 38 to 43°C range for warm receptors. The introduction of a cold stimulus to the skin increases the discharge rate for the cold receptors and decreases the discharge for the warm receptors. A warm stimulus causes the converse.[14,15,17] This overlapping of cold, warm, and pain nerve endings explains the paradoxical perception that the temperature extremes of icy cold and burning hot are almost alike.[5,15]

Thermal sensory perception is influenced by: (1) the area of stimulation, (2) the temperature gradiant, and (3) the duration of exposure. In the temperature range of 28 to 32°C differences of 1° should be perceived. In the cold range, the differential may increase to as high as 10°. In the warm range, a 5° difference should be distinguished.[19]

INTEGUMENT

The skin plays a major role in thermoregulation and the body's response to locally applied heat or cold. The eccrine glands, thermoreceptors, and hair follicles, all located in the skin, are actively involved in the body's response to heat.

Also intimately related to the control of body temperature is the extensive blood supply to the skin, which is arranged in two systems. One serves the nutritive requirement and the other serves thermoregulation. A highly developed network of subpapillary plexuses of capillaries and venules, and in some areas of the body, arteriovenous anastomoses, are actively involved in thermoregulation.[5,20] These blood vessels, innervated by sympathetic nerve fibers, will dilate to increase heat loss or constrict to decrease heat loss. With maximal vasodilatation, blood flow to the skin may be increased *seven* times normal. This degree of vasodilatation places a great demand on cardiac output which is of vital concern in the treatment of elderly patients.

In conjunction with the skin, subcutaneous fat provides a layer of insulation to conserve core temperature. The percentage of water in skin tissue also influences thermal conductivity. The dry insulative surface of the epidermis has a fairly constant level of heat conduction, in contrast to deeper areas of skin which are more variable in conduction due to perfusion and water content.[21]

THERMOREGULATION OF ELDERLY PERSONS

Heat Stroke

Various physiological functions decline with age at differential rates. What seem to be small or insignificant losses become greater problems when they are integrated into a system such as thermoregulation.[3] This breakdown may eventually be fatal. Heat-related deaths and heat stroke among the elderly during hot and humid weather are well documented.[22–24]

Heat stroke is more common among the elderly population because the normal vasodilatation response and subsequent cardiovascular adjustments of increased cardiac output and respiratory rate are more sluggish. Among elderly patients, there are common diseases, medications, and special problems that may increase the risk of heat injury:[24]

Diuretics prevent volume expansion and thus limit cutaneous vasodilatation.

Anticholinergic agents inhibit sweating.

Parkinson's disease increases muscular work, and the medications used to treat this condition have atropine-like effects that impair sweating.

Dermatological diseases may be associated with decreased or absent sweating.

Spinal cord lesions may also impair temperature-induced sweating because of the pathways to the hypothalamus.

Bedridden patients may be unable to remove clothes or to increase voluntary fluid intake.

Sensation of thirst may decrease.

Heat Exhaustion

Heat exhaustion characterized by pallor, profuse sweating, vomiting, an urge to defecate, giddiness, and postural syncopy results from inadequate cardiovascular compensation to heat-induced vasodilatation. This condition is very similar to a typical vasovagal attack.[24]

Hypothermia

During the winter months, hypothermia, which is defined as rectal temperature below 35°C can cause death.[25] In addition to fatalities, increased hospitalization and concomitant illnesses have been related to hypothermia during cold weather,[25,26] because in some elderly persons the isothermal system is altered with age. In a national survey in Great Britain of persons living at home, Fox and colleagues reported that 10 percent of their subjects had core temperatures below 35.5°C.[27] These temperatures were recorded during winter months.

Thatcher reported a statistically significant difference of .5°C between mean oral temperatures of elderly persons taken during the summer and winter months. When compared to the norm of 37.3°C, both seasonal temperatures were significantly less than the norm. Another important question was raised about normal temperature for elderly persons because the mean temperature was 36.6°C but the range was nearly 1.7°C (96.29–99.23°F.)[29]

Among most independently living elderly persons, core temperature does not appear to be changed.[27,28] Collins and his colleagues reported urine temperatures in 147 elderly subjects of 36.33°C in the morning and 36.56°C in the afternoon. Four years later, there were no changes in mean urine temperatures in 47 of the same subjects (age range 69 to 90 years). In contrast, skin temperature of the hand was 31.29 and 33.08°C in the morning and afternoon, respectively. Four years later, these temperatures were significantly lower at 30.31 and 31.96°C.[27] These data indicate that circadian rhythms influence core and skin temperatures in elderly persons as in younger persons.

As shown in Figure 5-1, skin temperature in elderly persons as well as in younger persons is dependent on the measured body part, with the periphery being cooler. Howell reported mean temperatures of 35.8°C, with a range of 32.4 to 37.8°C for the groin; and 26.8°C, with a range of 20.0 to 37.2°C for the left toe in 104 hospitalized women with an age range of 61 to 100 years. He interpreted these data as indicating that the circulatory status in some elderly persons remains relatively unchanged whereas others are in danger of having inadequate arterial circulation, as evidenced by the wide range of skin temperature.[30,31]

Core temperature may be lower because basal metabolism declines after the age of 30 years at an average rate of 1.66 calories per meter per hour per decade. In other words, basal metabolism decreases from ~38 cal/m/h at 30 years of age to ~30 cal/m/h at 80 years of age. This amounts to a decrease of only 15 percent; however, basal metabolism is a principle source of body heat. Regardless of this age-related decline, Shock noted that some persons in the ninth decade of life had basal metabolic rates as high as those of the 40-year-old subjects. Additionally, Shock reported that the fall in basal metabolism reflected a loss of metabolizing tissue and not a loss of heat-productive ability of the remaining tissues.[3]

Faulty Thermoregulation

Dilman hypothesized that the role of the hypothalamus in homeostatic regulation is a major factor in age-related declines,[32] stating that with increasing age the hypothalamus becomes less sensitive to the physiological feedback and consequently is less able to maintain the stability of the internal environment of the body. Processes such as increased body weight, increased serum cholesterol, and decreased glucose tolerance ensue; subsequently, diseases result.

The hypothalamic thermostat is the principle control center for regulating the body's response to ambient, locally applied, and internal temperature gradients. Many investigators have attributed the increased rate of heat stroke, hypothermia, and climate-related deaths among the aged population to faulty thermoregulation.[26–28]

Not only the hypothalamic thermostat and basal metabolic rate but also the overall reactivity of the autonomic nervous system declines with age, altering skin hydration and circulation in turn.[33] The vasomotor system is less responsive to warming and cooling[27] and the normal transient bursts of vasoconstrictor activity are reduced.[34] It is unclear whether or not thermoreceptors in the skin are altered; however Collins and co-workers reported significant differences in thermal perception. Young subjects could perceive mean temperature differences on the finger of 0.8 and 0.9°C for cold and warm stimuli. In contrast, the older group responded to differences of 2.3 and 2.5°C, respectively.[27] Because cold receptors are dependent on a good oxygen supply, Collins and Exton-Smith reasoned that decreased circulatory supply may decrease perception of cold because of the vulnerability of cold receptors to hypoxia.[34] Although not testing for thermoreceptor impulses, Watts reported that his group of 18 elderly women living independently (age range 74 to 86 years) were able to perceive environmental cold and cold discomfort accurately.[35]

Skin atrophy is another factor that may reduce the efficiency of thermoregulation. Atrophied skin is less able to protect against heat loss. The marked reduction in skin circulation, especially the vertical capillary groups in the dermal papillae, has a deleterious effect on hair bulbs, eccrine, apocrine, and sebaceous glands.[36]

Hellon and Lind compared sweat gland activity in 10 young men (ages 18 to 23 years) and 10 older men (ages 44 to 57 years). They reported that the mean time of sweating onset in a hot room was 15 minutes for the young group and 29 minutes for the older group and that the older group had a lower number of operative sweat glands.[37] Because the older subjects had lower skin temperatures at the onset, this decreased sweating response may have been modified by lower starting skin temperature, as reported by Nadel and colleagues.[10] Collins and associates also reported that their older subjects showed a decreased sweating response to environmental heating.[27]

In contrast, Drinkwater et al reported no significant differences between 10 young women (mean age 38.4 ± 2.1 years) and 10 postmenopausal women (mean age 57.7 ± 1.2 years) in time of onset and threshold temperature for sweating. They found that the sweat rate was related to VO_{max} and not to age.[38] Similarly Yousef and colleagues found that sweating rates were not affected by age in desert heat. In their study, each of the subjects walked for 1 hour at 40 percent of aerobic capacity. Changes in the mean temperature during the walk were similiar in all age groups. The increase in rectal temperature was similar in all age groups. These investigators suggested that the key to the successful regulatory response was the control of exercise at a level of 40 percent aerobic capacity.[39]

Other influences on thermal perception and temperature regulation may be:

1. A decreased ability to shiver.
2. Decreased muscle mass.
3. Painful arthritic joints which may discourage increased physical activity as a response to cold.[34]
4. Medication.[24,40] In a recent study in Sweden, 44 percent of the patients taking antihypertensive drugs complained of cold hands and/or feet. Fifty-four percent of the patients using β-blocker medication suffered this problem as compared with 35 percent of the patients using diuretics alone. The investigators stated that the complaint of coldness could not be attributed solely to drugs.
5. Alcohol. Ingestion of alcohol is another detriment to thermoregulation. From 1972 to 1982, 48 percent of the exposure-related hypothermia deaths in the District of Columbia had blood ethanol levels >0.15 g/dL.[25]
6. Low income. Although not under physiological control, low income is another factor that encourages thermal insult because of fuel costs, lack of air conditioning, inadequate housing, and poor nutrition.[22,23,25–28,34,35]

SUMMARY

In summary, the control of body temperature is a sophisticated process involving most tissues of the body and especially the hypothalamus, the skin, the circulatory system, and the nervous system. Altered (faulty) thermoregulation is a serious problem, especially for elderly persons, and may lead to harmful effects and even death. The therapeutic application of heat or cold to a body part is not isolated from the impact of this sophisticated thermoregulatory system and the changes associated with advanced age. The following factors must be considered in the treatment of elderly patients:

1. Ambient temperature and humidity[27]
2. Alterations in core temperature[28]
3. Declines in basal metabolic rate[3]
4. Abasement of hypothalamic feedback system[32]
5. Reduction in autonomic and vasomotor responses[34]
6. Diminution of temperature gradient perception[26]
7. Atrophy of skin[36]
8. Degradation in the circulatory system[36]
9. Loss of sweat glands[37]
10. Decline in aerobic capacity[38]
11. Response to medications [24]

The therapist who treats elderly persons should understand these changes; however, it is essential to note that each patient is an individual and that the declines that occur in aging do not affect everyone similarly. Thus, not every aging patient will have a faulty thermoregulatory system.

THERMAL INJURY

Heat

In most therapeutic settings, when heat is applied to elderly persons precautions are taken to prevent a burn. These actions often include: extra layers of towel; reduced hydrocollator temperature; shorter treatment time, precautions to insure that the patient never lies on the hot pack; reduced intensity or non-use of ultrasound. These precautions appear to be justified, considering the data on burns among the elderly.

The incidence of hospitalization of persons with new burns is 27 in 100,000; however, for persons 75 to 79, 80 to 85, and ≥85 years of age, the incidence increases to 28, 37, and 41 persons per 100,000, respectively.[41] In Linn's sample of 1,297 patients who were admitted to 73 different hospitals for burns, the >65-year-old group was more likely to suffer a severe burn and more likely to develop complications. This was attributed to declining psychomotor skills, skin atrophy, and a decline in epidermal cell proliferation. In this sample, 24 percent of the older burn victims died, as compared with 1, 5, and 6 percent for the respective age groups of <15, 15 to 44, and 45 to 64 years of age.[42]

Baptiste and Feck reported on 793 hot liquid burns that occurred in upstate New York during 1974 to 1975. Tap water was the cause of 196 or 24.7 percent of these burns; 50 percent of these burns occurred in toddlers and 27 percent occurred in persons >60 years of age. Among the elderly victims, the burns resulted from falling or losing consciousness in the bath or shower. Although the temperatures that caused these burns were not recorded, the investigators advocated that household water temperature be reduced to 48.9°C (120°F).[43]

This recommendation is based on the extensive work by Moritz and Henriques, who studied the relationship of time and temperature to cutaneous burns.[44] These investigators applied heated water or oil directly to the skin of human subjects; ages were not specified. Exposure to water or oil at 44°C for 6 hours led to complete epidermal necrosis. At 48°C, 15 minutes of exposure caused a second- or third-degree burn. At 51°C, only 2 minutes of exposure yielded a thermal injury of epidermal necrosis. A first-degree reaction without loss of epidermal tissue occurred at 30 seconds at 53°C. A 5-second exposure at 60°C of heated oil led to complete epidermal necrosis. This association between temperature and duration is important because the recommended temperature of the thermostatically controlled, popularly used hydrocollator unit is 71 to 80°C, and the treatment length is 20 to 30 minutes.[45,46]

Moritz and Henriques compared their results in humans with time/temperature thresholds in pig skin and found no quantitative difference in the susceptibility to thermal injury[44]; therefore, the following investigations were conducted on pigs. No transepidermal necrosis was found at exposures of 7 minutes at 49°C or at 2 minutes at 51°C, but all exposures of 9 minutes at 49°C and 4 minutes at 51°C caused epidermal necrosis. These results represented burn thresholds of skin at these temperature and time exposures. At 49°C, the physiological characteristics of the skin and dermal capillaries were sufficient to prevent irreversible damage at 7 minutes but not at 9 minutes of exposure.

To investigate the extent to which ischemia may increase the vulnerability of the epidermis to burns, the researchers applied water to pig skin at 80 mm pressure, an amount sufficient to impair blood flow. With this pressure on the surface of the skin during the exposure of heat, there were no burns at a 7-minute time period at 49°C or at a 2-minute exposure at 51°C. The researchers indicated that the application of pressure sufficient to collapse the superficial dermal capillaries did not cause appreciable augmentation in the vulnerability of the epidermis to thermal injury.

Moritz and Henriques also investigated the cumulative effects of heat application. Using the threshold concept that no injury occurred at 49°C if the duration of exposure was less than 9 minutes, they applied heat in repeated episodes for a cumulative exposure of 9 minutes. Three exposures of 3 minutes each with intervals between exposures from 3 to 24 minutes all led to complete and irreversible epidermal necrosis. They reasoned that although visually recognizable necrosis did not occur after the first or second 3-minute exposure, a certain amount of epidermal injury occurred during the subthreshold exposure. A cumulative effect led to the damage unless there was an interval of ≤24 minutes between heat applications. If the interval was >24 minutes between 3-minute applications of heat, the tissue had an opportunity to recover from the epidermal injury sustained during the first 3 minutes.[44]

The above data are most pertinent because they demonstrate the integral relationship between time and temperature of safe and unsafe exposures to heat; and thus, therapeutically, we must consider the following.

1. Although heat is not applied for 6 hours in the clinic, patients do use heating pads for long periods of time and some even sleep on them. In this case, temperature must be <44°C.

2. Seldom is heat applied repeatedly in a therapeutic setting, but patients treat themselves repeatedly throughout the day.

3. When applied to a patient, moist heat packs must be properly secured so that not even a corner of a pack can be juxtaposed to a patient's skin. This unfortunate situation may result if a patient moves around or places his hand under the cover or towel. At the recommended starting temperature, irreversible tissue damage occurs in seconds.

4. Experimentally induced ischemia did not lead to increased burns; however, one must not forego good clinical judgment when applying heat to any patient, regardless of skin or circulatory status.

Cold

Cold application, like heat, has potential deleterious effects. Local cooling of a body part can lower core body temperature, in which case older persons are at greater risk.[26,34] Acute red wheals, indicative of possible skin injury, may occur at a temperature as high as 18°C.[47] Temperatures below 10°C cause pain, weakness, loss of fine motor ability, and eventual numbness.[47-49] Obvious tissue damage ensues at temperatures of ≥10°C. The freezing point of human fingers is between − .53 and − .65°C.[50] Like heat, duration and temperature are important. At 1.9°C no irreversible tissue damage occurs if cold is applied for 7 minutes; after 11½ minutes, however, hyperemia and tenderness results and lasts for several days. Repeated exposures cause blistering of the skin.[50]

Another systemic effect that must be considered when using cryotherapy is the cold pressor response, first described by Hines and Brown.[51] They found that when a supine subject placed a hand in 4°C water for 1 minute, the blood pressure measured in the opposite arm was elevated. Hypertensive subjects showed a large or hyperreactive response, which was interpreted to be characteristic of essential hypertension or a predisposition to it. More recently, it has been shown that the cold pressor response is mediated by sensory perception of cold-induced pain and not by essential hypertension.[52,53] Regardless of the nature of the elevation of blood pressure, one must be aware that blood pressure is likely to increase as a result of cold application of ≤15°C.[52] The colder the modality, the greater the increase in blood pressure. Wolfe reported respective elevations of systolic and diastolic pressures of 7 and 2 mmHg in the involved fingers of a hemiplegic patient and of 60 and 44 mmHg in the patient's uninvolved hand.[53]

DESIRED THERAPEUTIC EFFECTS OF HEAT AND COLD

In therapeutic settings, superficial heat is commonly applied with heating pads, moist heat packs, paraffin baths, hydrotherapy, and infrared. Other modalities such as short-wave diathermy, microwave diathermy, and ultrasound energy forms are converted to deep heat as they pass through the body's tissues.[45] The principal desired effects of heat include increases in blood flow and extensibility of collagen, as well as decreases in pain, spasm, and extracellular exudates.[45,46,54] The reasons to apply heat are no different for young or old persons; however, the precautions to heat applications are more common for geriatric patients. The rationale for precautions for using heat with the elderly patient may include: impaired circulation, confusion, open wounds, inflammation, infection, decreased sensory perception, fractures, implants, and poor medical status.

Cryotherapy is commonly applied with cold packs, ice massage, ice packs, cold water baths, or ethyl chloride spray. It is used for brief periods to facilitate muscle reflex activity and for longer periods up to 20 minutes to reduce spasticity. Although cold application increases pain by firing cold pain receptors,[14,17,52] it is used to reduce pain as well.[48,49] Precautions to using cold as a therapeutic stimulus include impaired circulation; confusion; open wounds; prolonged use which increases inflammation, decreased sensory perception; low core body temperature; hypertension; and poor medical status. A patient's aversion to cold may also preclude the use of cryotherapy even when it is indicated.

THERAPEUTIC APPLICATION OF HEAT IN A GERIATRIC SETTING

Very little clinical research has been done to determine the heating response in elderly persons, even though this segment of the population suffers more than any other from conditions that respond favorably to heat treatment. From the model of progressive physiological decline described earlier in this chapter, the response to heat application should be different in older persons than in younger persons. However, aging is an individual process and must be recognized as such. It must not be confused with pathology. Also, age is a relative concept and must be carefully defined when used to describe certain physiological traits. Hellon and Lind made specific reference to sweat gland activity in younger persons 18 to 23 years of age and older persons 47 to 57 years of age.[37] Howell recorded nose-tip temperature in persons ranging in age from 57 to 98 years.[31] In the first study, the oldest subject was the same age as the youngest subject in the second study, and Howell's data covered four decades of life; all were grouped under aging.

MOIST HEAT, A PILOT STUDY

The effects of moist heat on skin temperature have been reported in four young subjects, ages 19 and 24. The temperature peaked at ~45°C after ~5 minutes of application.[55] In an earlier report, Lehmann and co-workers stated that skin temperature of the human thigh peaked after 8 to 10 minutes of hydrocollator application. The ages and sexes of the subjects were not specified.[56] Considering the age-related changes in circulation, nervous system, and skin, one must ask if the skin temperature response is the same in geriatric patients.

With this in mind, we conducted a pilot study to answer the following questions.[57] What are the skin temperature changes that occur during the application of moist heat in a clinical setting? Are these changes age-related?

Subjects

Forty-one volunteers were recruited from the neighborhood, retirement communities, and three nursing homes. Ages ranged from 7 to 94 years; there were 19 females and 22 males.

The hip and the lower back are body parts that are commonly treated with moist heat. Thus, we allowed the subjects to choose which body part was to receive the moist heat. The back was chosen by 29 subjects; 12 were treated on either hip. These body parts are usually treated in the supine, sitting, side-lying, and prone positions. Six subjects chose the supine position, 9 chose the sitting, 12 the side-lying, and 14 the prone position.

The sample was divided into a young group (mean age 29.2 years) and an older group (mean age 79.2 years). There were six females and 14 males in the young group, with an age range of 7 to 44 years, a difference of 37 years. The older group had 13 females and 8 males, with an age range of 59 to 94 years, a difference of 35 years.

Methods

An Orthotherm infrared gun (Orthion Corp, Costa Mesa, Calif) was used to record skin temperature at the greater trochanter and at the spinous process of L5. A standard-size hydrocollator pack (Chattanooga Corp, Chattanooga, Tenn) was wrapped in a commercially available terrycloth cover (Chattanooga) and applied for 20 minutes to the selected body part. Skin temperature measurements were made at pretest and at 1, 3, 5, 10, 15, and 20 minutes, at which time the pack was removed. Skin temperature was measured during the cooling phase at 1, 3, 5, 10, 15, 20, 30, and 40 minutes. All testing was done between 7:45 a.m. and 11:30 a.m.

Results

For the entire sample of 41 subjects, the mean starting skin temperature was 32.8°C and the mean maximal temperature was 42.4°C. An average of 10.1 minutes was required to reach maximum temperature. A significant negative

Table 5-1. Correlational Coefficients of Age, Time, and Temperatures

Factor	2	3	4	5	6	7	8	9
1. Age	.58[a]	.59[b]	.21	−.25	−.36[c]	.04	−.34[d]	.38[e]
2. Start room temperature	—	.86[a]	−.09	−.27	−.29	.15	−.16	.23
3. End room temperature	—	—	.01	−.02	−.16	.14	−.18	.35[f]
4. Start hydrocollator temperature	—	—	—	.37°	.51[a]	−.02	.03	.10
5. Start pack temperature	—	—	—	—	.56[h]	−.03	.15	−.15
6. End pack temperature	—	—	—	—	—	.16	.14	.04
7. Start skin temperature	—	—	—	—	—	—	−.11	.02
8. Max skin temperature	—	—	—	—	—	—	—	−.53[i]
9. Time to max								

[a] $P < 0.001$ [b] $P < .0004$ [c] $P < .03$
[d] $P < .02$ [e] $P < .01$ [f] $P < .05$
[g] $P < .003$ [h] $P < .0006$ [i] $P < .0003$

Table 5-2. Skin Temperature Changes with Moist Heat In Person 7 to 94 Years of Age

Age	N	Sex	SKTO °C	Max T °C	Time (min)	Comments
7	2	M, M	37.0	43.2	10,10	—
15	1	F	31.9	43.3	10	—
22	1	M	31.8	39.3	10	—
25	2	M, F	30.9	42.6	15,10	—
26	2	M, M	33.2	42.4	10,15	1 extra towel
28	1	M	33.4	44.8	10	2 extra towels
29	1	M	29.4	45.0	5	1 extra towel
30	1	M	32.5	42.2	5	—
33	2	F, M	32.4	44.3	5,10,3	1 towel each
34	2	F, M	32.9	43.1	5,10	—
37	1	F	35.1	42.6	10	—
42	1	M	31.7	41.8	10	1 extra towel
43	1	M	30.6	43.9	10	1 extra towel
44	2	M, F	29.8	42.4	10,5	1 extra towel
				43.0		
59	1	M	34.0		10	—
67	1	F	31.6	42.2	10	—
68	1	F	33.0	46.7	5	Back, supine
71	2	M, F	31.8	43.3	10,20	—
75	1	F	34.9	43.0	15	—
76	1	M	30.4	39.6	10	DJD hip
						4 extra towels BK
						amp, CVA,
77	1	M	30.9	44.1	3,5	DJD
78	3	F, F, M	34.6	40.7	10,10,5	—
						Hip fx,
79	2	F, F	35.0	42.5	10,10	Compression fx
81	1	M	33.7	44.9	10	1 extra towel
83	1	F	33.2	42.9	10,15	DJD
						Side-lying, no
87	1	F	33.9	40.1	10	sheet
90	2	M, F	32.2	40.7	10,20	Hip fx, hip fx
91	1	M	31.9	42.9	15	HNP
92	1	F	31.5	35.3	21	Hip fx, CVA
94	1	F	35.1	38.9	15	DJD
54.8	41	19F, 22 M	32.8	42.4	10.1	

In those age groups with more than one subject, the mean temperatures and each individual's time for maximal temperature are recorded. In several cases, a peak temperature was recorded at two separate times.

BK amp = below knee amputation
Fx = fracture
HNP = herniated nucleus pulposis
DJD = degenerative joint disease
CVA = cerebrovascular accident
SKTO = starting skin temperature

correlation was found between age and maximum skin temperature ($r = -.34$, $P < .02$). A significant positive correlation was found between age and maximum skin temperature ($r = -.38$; $P < .01$). Starting skin temperature and maximum temperature were negatively and insignificantly correlated ($r = -.11$). Maximum temperature was positively but insignificantly related to starting hot pack temperature ($r = .15$); and to ending hot pack temperature ($r = .14$). These data are presented in Tables 5-1 and 5-2.

When the young and old groups are compared, the starting skin temperatures were 32.5 and 33.1°C, respectively. The maximal skin temperatures were 43.0 and 41.8°C for the young and old groups. The times to maximum temperature were 8.7 minutes and 11.4 minutes for the young and old groups, respectively. When compared with an analysis of variance, these variables showed no statistically significant differences between the two groups.

Discussion

Statistically significant correlations between age and maximum temperature and time to maximum temperature indicated that as age increased the maximum skin temperature was lower and it took longer to reach maximum temperature (Table 5-1). This may have been influenced by several variables such as pathology, number of towels, and position. As can be seen in Table 5-2, none of the younger persons, compared to ~50 percent of the older persons, had pathological conditions that may have influenced the body's response to heat.

The first subject was a 78-year-old man who was treated in the side-lying position without a sheet wrapped around him to hold the pack against his body. In addition, two terry cloth pads were used, whereas all other subjects started with only one pad. The subject's initial skin temperature at the L5 spinous process was 34.4°C; he reached a peak skin temperature of only 36.8°C at 10 minutes. Not only the padding but also the position influenced these results.

Similarly, the 94-year-old subject was treated in the side-lying position without a sheet to hold the hot pack against her body. She was uncomfortable and unable to lie still; thus, the hot pack fell off her back onto the floor after the 5-minute measurement. At $12\frac{1}{2}$ minutes, she asked for a change in position from side-lying to sitting. These factors influenced the shape of the curve in Figure 5-3.

Skin temperature at the lateral malleolus was measured in several subjects as moist heat was applied to their hips. As can be seen in Figure 5-3, ankle skin temperature did not increase during heat application. No control was used to determine if loss of skin temperature would have been greater if no heat had been applied to the hip. The peripheral effects of proximal heat application need further study.

Several other important features are noted in Figure 5-3. First, an elevated skin temperature was maintained up to 40 minutes after cessation of heat application. Second, the starting skin temperature did not influence maximum skin temperature. As can be seen, the 7-year-old and the 33-year-old subjects started at different temperatures but peaked at nearly the same temperature.

As shown in Table 5-2, some of the older subjects also reached a maximum temperature at ~43°C. This may represent a physiological ceiling or threshold of comfort and safety. Nearly all the subjects who had skin temperatures >43.5°C asked for an extra towel. The work of Moritz and Henriques demonstrated that irreversible tissue damage occurred at 44°C when heat was ap-

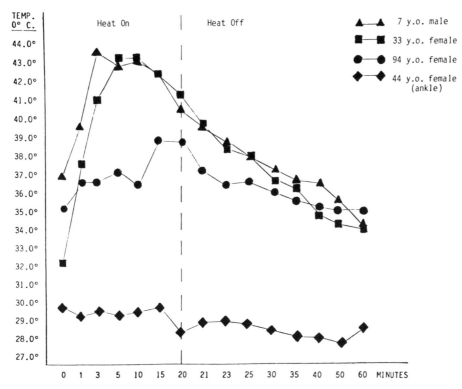

Fig. 5-3. Effect of moist heat packs on skin temperature.

plied to skin for 6 hours.[44] Zotterman suggested that the paradoxical sensation of heat and cold occurred just above 43.0°C.[15]

As can be seen in Figure 5-2, transient pain can be evoked by heat, at temperatures of 37 to 40°C; however, reproducible static pain results from temperatures in the 44 to 45°C range.[58]

Sherman and Robillard found a significant age-related increase in threshold of pain from a radiant heat stimulus.[59] For males 30 to 39 years of age, heat-provoked pain perception was 289.3 as compared with 328.0 mcal/s/cm² in the group 60 to 64 years of age. This was not found in our study. All of the older subjects, as did the younger subjects whose skin temperature went over 43.5°C, perceived the temperature as being too hot and asked for a towel. However, it was not our intent to measure pain perception.

During the application of moist heat, it is common practice to ask several times whether the patient is feeling heat and if it is too warm. In addition, the body part should be visually inspected so that normal hyperemia is noted and treatment is changed if the skin becomes angry, red, or mottled. We solicited from each patient at each time of measurement a verbal response indicating either no heat sensation, barely warm, warm, comfortably warm or hot, and hot. We also visually inspected the body area and recorded absence of color, slight pink color, bright red color, and mottling. We did not find these accepted clinical practices to correspond very well with skin temperatures as measured on the Orthotherm infrared gun. As expected, initially subjects felt warmth without redness but usually within 5 to 10 minutes after removal of heat, they felt no heat even though there was redness, and the skin temperature had not returned to pre test levels. It was not uncommon for the skin temperature to be elevated even 40 minutes after the hot pack was removed and to find slight to moderate hyperemia at the end of treatment.

Summary

1.   Older persons responded to moist heat as did younger persons.
2.   The positioning of the subjects, the method of moist heat application, and control of heat loss from the body and hot pack were more important than age in determining the change in skin temperature with moist heat.
3.   A physiologic ceiling for skin temperature with moist heat application appeared to be 42.5 to 43.5°C.
4.   The thermoregulatory capabilities and response to moist heat appeared to be maintained in our older sample. However, these results may not represent the entire population of older persons.

CONCLUSION

Age-related changes are reported in tissues and systems involved in temperature regulation and the body's response to heat and cold both locally and environmentally. These changes should be considered in treatment of elderly persons, although they will not be found in all geriatric patients. Indications and precautions for using heat/cold are not dissimilar to those for young persons; however, there are several special considerations. Medical conditions such as atherosclerotic cardiovascular disease or the use of certain drugs such as diuretics, anticholinergic agents, or antihypertensive drugs may render a patient less able to adjust to heat or cold application. A differentiation between the responses of the elderly population to the various types of heat or cold applications has not yet been thoroughly made. The efficacy of therapeutic interventions and the physiological responses to the application of thermal energy must be investigated if the care of the elderly is to be improved. Until then, the clinician must ask the following questions. What are the desired therapeutic effects of heat/cold? How can they best be applied? Are there any contraindications or precautions to treatment? Finally, the clinician must seek answers to these questions every day.

REFERENCES

1.   Orgel L: The maintenance of the accuracy of protein synthesis and its relevance to aging. Proc Natl Acad Sci USA 49:517, 1963
2.   Walton J: The role of limited cell replicative capacity in pathological age change. A review. Mech Age Dev 19:217, 1982

3. Shock N: Systems Integration. In Finch C, Hayflick L (eds): The Biology of Aging. VanNostrand Reinhold, New York, 1977
4. Hardy JD: The radiating power of human skin in the infra-red. Am J Physiol 127:454, 1939
5. Guyton AC: Basic Human Physiology Normal Function and Mechanisms of Disease. 2nd Ed. WB Saunders, Philadelphia 1977
6. Smith LW, Fay T: Temperature factors in cancer and embryonal cell growth. JAMA 113:653, 1939
7. Hardy JD: Physiology of temperature regulation. Physiol Rev 41:521, 1961
8. Jessen C, Feistkorn G, Nagel A: Temperature sensitivity of skeletal muscle in the conscious goat. J Appl Physiol 54:880, 1983
9. Gisolfi C, Wenger CB: Temperature regulation during exercise: old concepts, new concepts. In Terjung RL (ed): Exercise and Sport Sciences Reviews. Vol. 12. p. 339 Collamore Press, Lexington, Mass, 1984
10. Nadel E, Bullard R, Stolwijk J: Importance of skin temperature in the regulation of sweating. J Appl Physiol 31:80, 1971
11. Bini G, Hagbarth K, Hynninen P, Wallin B: Thermoregulatory and rhythm generating mechanisms governing the sudomotor and vasoconstrictor outflow in human cutaneous nerves. J Physiol 306:537, 1980
12. Ganong WF: Review of Medical Physiology. Lange Medical, Los Altos, Calif, 1969
13. Gagge AP, Stevens JC: Thermal sensitivity and comfort. In Kenshalo D (ed): The Skin Senses. Charles C. Thomas, Springfield, Ill, 1968
14. Hensel H: Thermoreceptors. Annu Rev Physiol 36:233 1974
15. Zotterman Y: Special senses: Thermal receptors. Annu Rev Physiol 15:357, 1953
16. Kibler R, Nathan T: A note on warm and cold spots. Neurology 10:874, 1960
17. Hardy J, Stolwijk J, Hoffman D: Pain following step increase in skin temperature. In Kenslow D (ed): The Skin Senses. Charles C Thomas, Springfield, Ill, 1968
18. Neisser U: Temperature thresholds for cutaneous pain. J Appl Physiol 14:368, 1959
19. Victor M, Adams R: Disorders of sensation. In Wintrobe M, Thorn G, Adams R, et al (eds): 142–147: Harrison's Principles of Internal Medicine. 6th Ed. McGraw Hill, New York, 1970
20. Ham A: Histology. 7th Ed. JB Lippincott, Philadelphia, 1974
21. Sekins KM, Emery AF: Thermal science for physical medicine. In Lehmann J, DeLatour B (eds): Therapeutic Heat and Cold. 3rd Ed. Williams & Wilkins, Baltimore, 1982
22. Morbidity and Mortality Weekly Report: Medical Examiner Summer Mortality Surveillance U.S., 1979–1981. p. 336. Vol 31. No. 25. July 2, 1982
23. Levine J: Heat stroke in the aged. Am J Med 47:251, 1969
24. Wheeler M: Heat stroke in the elderly. Med Clin North Am: 60(6):1289, 1976
25. Morbidity and Mortality Weekly Report. Exposure Related Hypothermia Deaths— District of Columbia, 1972–1982. p. 669. Vol. 31. No. 50. Dec. 24, 1982
26. Rango N: Old and cold: hypothermia in the elderly. Geriatrics 35:93, 1980
27. Collins K, Dore C, Exton-Smith A, et al: Accidental hypothermia and impaired temperature homeostasis in the elderly. Br Med J 1:353, 1977
28. Fox R, Woodward P, Exton-Smith A, et al: Body temperatures in the elderly: a national study of physiological, social, and environmental conditions. Br Med J 1:200, 1973
29. Thatcher R: 98.6°F. What is normal? J Gerontol Nurs 9:23, 1983
30. Howell T: Skin temperature gradient in the lower extremities of old women. Exp Gerontol 17:65, 1982

31. Howell TH: Nose tip temperature in the aged. Exp Gerontol 15:135, 1980
32. Dilman V: Age-associated elevation of hypothalmic threshold to feedback control, and its role in development, aging, and disease. Lancet 1:1211, 1971
33. Thompson L, Marsh G: Psychophysiological studies of aging. p. 112. In Eisdorfer C, Lawton M (eds): The Psychology of Adult Development and Aging. American Psychological Association Press, Washington DC, 1973
34. Collins K, Exton-Smith A: Thermal Homeostasis in old Age. J Am Geriatr Soc 31:519, 1983
35. Watts A: Hypothermia in the aged: a study of the role of cold sensitivity. Environ Res 5:119, 1971
36. Gilchrest B: Age-related changes in skin. p. 85 In Cape R, Coe R, Rossman I (eds): Fundamentals of Geriatric Medicine, Raven Press, New York, 1983
37. Hellon R, Lind A: Observations on the activity of sweat glands with special reference to the influence of aging. J Physiol 133:132, 1956
38. Drinkwater B, et al: Sweating sensitivity and capacity of women in relation to age. J Appl Physiol 53:671, 1982
39. Yousef M, Bedi J, Loucks A, et al: Thermoregulatory responses to desert heat: age, race and sex. J Gerontol 39:406, 1984
40. Feleke E, Lyngstam O, Rastam L, et al: Complaints of cold extremities among patients on antihypertensive treatment. Acta Med Scand 213:381, 1983
41. Feck G, Baptiste MS, Tate C Jr: An Epidemiologic Study of Burn Injuries and Strategies for Prevention. Center for Disease Control, Atlanta, Ga, 1978
42. Linn B: Age differences in the severity and outcome of burns. J Am Geriatr Soc 28:118, 1980
43. Baptiste M, Feck G: Preventing tap water burns. Am J Public Health 70:727, 1980
44. Moritz A, Henriques F Jr., Studies of thermal injury. II. The importance of time and surface temperature in the causation of cutaneous burns. Am J Pathol 23:695, 1947
45. Lehmann J, DeLateur B: Therapeutic heat. In Lehmann J, DeLateur B (eds): Therapeutic Heat and Cold. 3rd Ed. Williams & Wilkins, Baltimore, 1982
46. Millard JB: Conductive heating. In Licht S (ed): Therapeutic Heat and Cold. 2nd Ed. Elizabeth Licht, New Haven, Conn, 1965
47. Lewis T: Observations on some normal and injurious effects of cold upon the skin and underlying tissues. Br Med J 2:795, 1941
48. Licht S: Local cryotherapy. In Licht S (ed): Therapeutic Heat and Cold. 2nd ed. Elizabeth Licht, New Haven, Conn, 1965
49. Lehmann J, DeLateur B: Cryotherapy. In Lehman J, DeLateur B (eds): Therapeutic Heat and Cold 3rd Ed. Williams & Wilkins, Baltimore, 1982
50. Keatinge W, Cannon P: Freezing point of human skin. Lancet 1:11, 1960
51. Hines E, Brown G: A standard test for measuring the variability of blood pressure. Its significance as an index of the prehypertensive state. Ann Intern Med 7:209, 1933–1934
52. Wolf S, Hardy J: Studies on pain. Observations on pain due to local cooling and on factors involved in the "cold pressor" effect. J Clin Invest 20:521, 1941
53. Wolff H: The mechanism and significance of the cold pressor response. Q J Med 20:261, 1951
54. Fischer E, Solomon S: Physiological responses to heat and cold. In Licht S (ed): Therapeutic Heat and Cold. 2nd ed. Elizabeth Licht, New Haven, Conn 1965
55. Lehmann J, Stonebridge J, deLateur B, et al: Temperatures in human thighs after hot pack treatment followed by ultrasound. Arch Phys Med Rehabil 59:472, 1978

56. Lehmann J, Silverman D, Baum B, et al: Temperature distributions in the human thigh. Produced by infrared, hot pack and microwave applications. Arch Phys Med Rehabil 47:291, 1966
57. Kauffman T, Nwaobi O: Effects of age on skin temperature changes with moist heat. (submitted for publication)
58. Hardy J, Stolwijk J: Tissue temperature and thermal pain. In De Reuck A, Knight J (eds): Touch, Heat and Pain. Churchill, London, 1966
59. Sherman ED, Robillard E: Sensitivity to pain in relationship to age. J Am Geriatr Soc 12:1037, 1964

APPENDIX 5-1

Temperature Scales

Fahrenheit	Centigrade
170.0	76.7
150.0	65.6
140.0	60.0
135.0	57.2
130.0	54.4
125.0	51.7
120.0	48.9
115.0	46.1
110.0	43.3
105.0	40.6
100.0	37.8
98.6	37.0
97.0	36.1
96.0	35.5
95.0	35.0
94.0	34.4
92.0	33.3
90.0	32.2
88.0	31.1
85.0	29.4
80.0	26.6
75.0	23.8
70.0	21.1
60.0	15.6
50.0	10.0
40.0	4.4
32.0	0.0
30.0	−1.1

To convert Centigrade to Fahrenheit: $F = C\frac{9}{5} + 32$; to convert Fahrenheit to Centigrade, $C = \frac{5}{9}(F - 32)$.

6 | Wheelchair Needs of the Disabled

Susan C. Hallenborg

Because of an increase in susceptibility to illness and disability in older age,[1] the elderly represent a large percentage of wheelchair users. The characteristics of specific disabling conditions dictate the wheelchair needs of any wheelchair-dependent person, but the elderly require special consideration; that is, the wheelchair must compensate for age-related limitations as well as the primary disability. Visual loss, hearing loss, reduction in dexterity and coordination, changes in mental status, and postural distortion may all confound the disability status of the elderly patient.[1]

Anyone who spends a significant amount of time in a wheelchair must be carefully evaluated for appropriate fit to provide maximal comfort and function. The wheelchair can be most effectively prescribed if thought of as two separate systems, the seating system and the mobility system. Historically, the major concerns were choosing the appropriate method of propulsion, whether manual, power, or passive, and providing an appropriately fitting seat and back. Supportive seating components such as a firm seat or lateral supports were only prescribed after problems developed and rarely were considered at the time of initial prescription. However, clinicians are becoming increasingly aware that correct size and a good cushion may not be enough for all patients.[2] Carefully prescribed seating and mobility systems maximize potential for independent function in mobility and many activities of daily living (ADL),[3] ultimately benefiting both patient and caregivers.

This chapter is designed to introduce the reader to the basic principles of wheelchair prescription for the elderly. Emphasis is given to evaluation procedures and low technology, commercially available solutions to seating and mobility problems commonly seen among the disabled elderly.

THE WHEELCHAIR

The goals of the prescription wheelchair are to (1) correct flexible, existing postural problems; (2) accommodate fixed or structural orthopedic problems; and (3) compensate for loss or absence of function in order to promote a maximal level of independence. The adult with acute temporary disability (e.g., lower extremity fracture) generally has no need for special attention to correct or accommodate postural or structural orthopedic problems. The wheelchair is needed only to compensate for temporary loss of the ability to ambulate. A properly prescribed wheelchair, however, may allow the otherwise bedridden patient to remain active and independent in ADL, resulting in prevention of the debilitating effects of bedrest and inactivity. It is important to make clear to the alert and oriented patient the purpose of using a wheelchair temporarily and the expected length of use, since the patient may have unspoken fears of long-term use.

The presence of a permanent mobility impairment dictates the need for individualized wheelchair prescription[4] that meets all three of the stated goals. The wheelchair, with its seating and mobility components, should be considered an orthotic device. It should be carefully prescribed to maximize comfort, safety, and function.

In addition to compensation for the primary disability, the wheelchair can assist in the prevention of secondary disability. Problems which may develop as a result of lack of attention to primary disability include skin problems, joint contractures, and disuse atrophy.[1] Attention to prevention of secondary disabilities will help to minimize the need for care by family or staff and maximize the user's potential for independence and heightened self-esteem.

The dangers of a poorly prescribed wheelchair are numerous. Hartigan[5] describes three common wheelchair seating problems resulting from misuse of the standard adult "transport" wheelchair. The standard chair with its sling style seat and back is designed for convenient, temporary transportation and is *not* appropriate for long-term sitting. The patient who is confined to this style of chair for any length of time will most assuredly demonstrate symptoms of wheelchair seating problems.

The most common early symptom of a seating problem is discomfort. Nursing home patients may express this discomfort by frequent requests to "go back to bed." Postural problems may either be the cause or result of discomfort. Forward slouching, leaning to one side, or hanging on to one armrest may be observed. These postural problems may be corrected when they first occur, but will undoubtedly result in structural orthopedic problems if allowed to persist. If minor symptoms of seating problems are ignored, a more serious symptom, skin breakdown, may develop. Early recognition and correction of seating problems will prevent the occurrence of this and other unnecessary secondary complications.

Symptomatic treatment of seating problems is, unfortunately, a common clinical practice. Foam cushion "cutouts" for weight relief and/or bedrest may be necessary to heal skin breakdown, but this symptomatic approach to treat-

ment alone is not enough. If the underlying cause for the symptom is not identified and treated, the patient is left at risk for recurrence of the problem. The
underlying causes can only be identified through a thorough assessment of the
patient's seating and mobility needs.

EVALUATION OF WHEELCHAIR NEEDS

To what degree, if any, will the wheelchair need to compensate for loss
or absence of function, to correct flexible postural problems, or to accommodate fixed structural orthopedic problems? These questions can be answered
only after a careful assessment. The wheelchair evaluation begins with assessment of sitting posture. The sitting assessment should be conducted with
the patient seated in a chair with a firm but padded seat and back. The seat
and back should be placed at an angle as close to 90° as possible. The examiner
should then compare the patient's posture to an optimal or "ideal" sitting
posture. Ideal posture is outlined in Table 6-1 as a frame of reference.

When deviations from optimal alignment or symmetry are noted, the examiner must determine the source of the problem. Is it a limitation of motion,
a structural problem such as a leg length discrepancy, extensor spasticity, tonic
reflex activity, or a combination of problems? Each contributing problem must
be identified separately before appropriate solutions can be provided. Evalu-
ations of musculoskeletal and neuromuscular systems are generally done si-

Table 6-1. "Ideal" Postural Alignment in Sitting

Body Segment	Desired Posture	Benefit(s)
Pelvis	Slight anterior tilt, no lateral tilt, no rotation	Results in more stable position of spine Shifts weight-bearing to ischial tuberosities
Hips	Flexion ⩾90°, slight abduction, and slight external rotation	Helps maintain pelvic posture Provides wide stable base of support
Knees	Flexion near 90°	Minimizes stress on hamstrings
Feet	Neutral, plantargrade	Maintains functional range of motion
Spine	"Plumb-line" posture with slight lumbar lordosis, slight thoracic kyphosis, and slight cervical lordosis	Minimizes stress on trunk musculature Mechanically stable position for spine
Shoulder girdle	Neutral protraction/retraction	Minimizes stress to neck and upper back musculature Functional position for upper extremities
Head	Midline, vertical; eyes horizontal	Optimizes visual motor and oral motor functions
Upper extremities	Relaxed on armrests or in lap	Frees patient for propulsion or other functional task

multaneously, in a clinically relevant fashion, but are discussed separately here for the sake of clarity.

Musculoskeletal Assessment

The assessment always begins at the potential source of more distal problems, the base of support. The pelvis and lower extremities comprise the base of support in sitting. The position of these body segments will influence posture and function in the trunk, head, and upper extremities. Thus, identification of seating problems should always begin here. Correction or accommodation of problems at the base of support often negates the need for more distal correction or support.

Alignment and flexibility are assessed in supine and sitting positions. In the supine position, the pelvis is examined for flexibility in the frontal plane (lateral tilting), the horizontal plane (rotation), and the sagittal plane (anterior and posterior tilting). Sitting posture is examined for deviations from the ideal alignment illustrated in Figure 6-1. The weight-bearing forces should be borne as equally as possible to avoid excessive pressure to any one area. This is achieved with a neutrally positioned pelvis with no lateral tilting (obliquity) and both sides of the buttocks evenly seated against the backrest. It is most important that there is a slight anterior pelvic tilt, so that weight is borne on the ischial tuberosities. The ideal lower extremity position requires 90° of hip

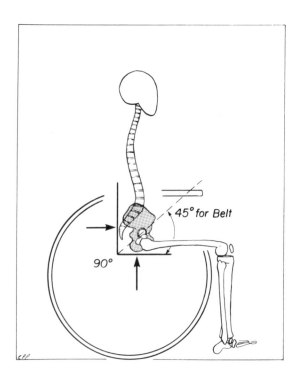

Fig. 6-1. Optimal pelvic alignment achieved with three-point pressure system.

flexion, slight abduction (modesty must be considered, and the older woman patient may need a lap robe or other draping to feel at ease in this position) and external rotation of the hips, 90° of knee flexion, and a neutral ankle position (no dorsiflexion/plantarflexion or inversion/eversion). Any asymmetry from right to left should be noted, since discrepancies must be accommodated in the seating system to achieve the desired positioning.

Once the pelvis and lower extremities have been positioned properly, attention is shifted to the upper body. Flexibility, alignment, and symmetry of the spine are examined in supine, sidelying, and sitting positions. As illustrated in Figure 6-1, the ideal alignment of the spine is that of a lumbar lordosis, a slight thoracic kyphosis, and a slight cervical lordosis. There is, of course, no scoliosis, and the posterior aspect of the trunk rests symmetrically and comfortably on the backrest. Alignment of the spine depends first on achievement of the ideal pelvic position described above. Slight anterior tilt of the pelvis helps mechanically to achieve the desired "extended" position of the spine, limiting the degree of flexibility between vertebrae, especially in the directions of lateral flexion and rotation.

More often than not, the older adult will not have the complete flexibility needed to achieve the desired ideal sitting posture. Therefore, the most crucial aspect of the musculoskeletal assessment is to determine to what degree deviations are fixed or flexible. To ensure comfort and support, accommodation of problems must be provided if deviations cannot be corrected by pelvic position or external support. This concept is further discussed later in this chapter.

Neuromuscular Assessment

Components of the wheelchair seating system may be used to compensate for muscle weakness, abnormal muscle tone, the effects of tonic reflex patterns, and/or delay or absence of righting or equilibrium reactions. Thus, the thorough neuromuscular evaluation is designed to identify any problems in these areas.

Objective assessment of strength is described in detail elsewhere.[6] Generally speaking, a gross assessment of strength is sufficient for wheelchair evaluation. Of primary concern are trunk control, head control, and upper extremity function. External postural supports for the trunk and head are needed if the patient is unable to maintain alignment and balance voluntarily while propelling the wheelchair (or while being propelled if a passive mobility system is used). Sitting balance must be able to be maintained *without upper extremity support*. The upper extremities will not be available for functional activities while the patient is sitting if they are used to maintain an upright posture. Postural support would be better provided with seating system components. Upper extremity control is important in choosing the method of wheelchair propulsion (ie, manual, powered, or passive), but many additional factors are of aid in making decisions about the mobility system. (See section on functional assessment.)

Resting muscle tone is assessed with a quick passive stretch of involved muscle groups. Although muscle tone assessment remains a subjective judgment, it is an important component of the wheelchair evaluation. Grading can be assigned as normal, hypotonic, hypertonic, or fluctuating. Any abnormality can be graded as minimal, moderate, or marked. The effect of voluntary effort on resting muscle tone is also noted, since this is the tonal state more likely to be experienced by a patient while actively using a wheelchair. For example, if extensor tone increases with voluntary effort, measures to inhibit this response can be provided in the seating system. It is important to identify an effective control for undesirable posturing. The therapist should observe whether changing the patient's body-part to body-part positioning (e.g., increasing hip flexion angle) rather than changing the body-in-space position (e.g., tilting the seating system back on the wheelchair frame) is more effective.

Finally, reflex testing is conducted to determine presence and strength of primitive reflex patterns as well as higher level righting and equilibrium responses. Any delays or absence of postural reactions will need compensation from the seating system. Techniques of reflex assessment are described elsewhere.[7,8]

Medical Assessment

Medical problems, both chronic and acute, must be identified and taken into account in the wheelchair prescription. Life expectancy as well as functional prognosis need consideration. If status is expected to improve or worsen, the prescriber should consider chair rental or purchase of wheelchair with parts which allow for change.[3]

Acute medical problems may influence seating and mobility needs, at least temporarily. A urinary tract infection, for example, may create a significant increase in spasticity in a person with spinal cord injury. However, this is usually a temporary problem, so it rarely warrants special provisions in the definitive wheelchair prescription.

Chronic medical problems have impact on the decision-making process. A patient with bilateral above-knee amputation may have sufficient strength to propel a manual wheelchair, but cardiovascular impairment may limit endurance. Purchase or rental of a powered wheelchair may be a more appropriate choice.

Functional Assessment

An appropriate wheelchair prescription should, in some way, improve functional ability, never reduce it. The only way to ensure that functional independence is enhanced or maintained is to consider all aspects of the person's lifestyle when determining the seating and mobility prescription. Self-care skills, recreational or leisure time activities, and family/community participation are all important considerations. If the wheelchair user is dependent on others for travel or care, the caregiver's abilities and concerns must be considered.

Physical strength and endurance are key determinants to the method of propulsion chosen. An additional concern in the elderly is perceptual function. The elderly may have exaggerated perceptions of speed, resulting in fear of independent mobility even though the goal may be physically possible. Fear-reducing measures, such as training in limited environments and techniques to reduce maximal speed of powered chairs, should be taken. The therapist must remember that independence can improve the patient's quality of life and self-esteem and should be provided wherever possible.[9] As Shinnar[10] points out, "Independence is the key to self-respect and dignity."

Current Equipment

The wheelchair that is currently being used by the patient should be judged for its appropriateness. A note should be made of any modifications or accessories that have been tried and the outcome of those attempts. Homemade adaptations are the most obvious indicator of the user's perceptions of personal needs.

Prosthetics or orthotics should be taken into account, especially if they interface in some way with the wheelchair. Use of a unilateral knee-ankle-foot orthosis or above-knee lower extremity prosthesis will create an asymmetry in sitting posture and will require accommodation in the seating system. If the device is only used part-time, the seating system should be designed to accommodate either situation.

Emotional and Mental Status

Inability to propel the wheelchair may be the result of fear or simple lack of desire to move. Seating problems such as slouching postures may be the result of sadness or loss of self-esteem. It is only through a careful assessment that the underlying causes for apparent seating and mobility problems can be determined. Solomon[11] outlines a guide for mental status examination of the elderly.

PRINCIPLES OF PROBLEM SOLVING

Identify Goals, Objectives, and Solutions

A strategic approach to problem solving will ensure that all concerns identified in the evaluation are addressed. The first step in the problem-solving hierarchy is identification of an overall goal for wheelchair use (eg, part-time transportation, full-time compensation for mobility problems). The next steps

include evaluation of medical, functional, and personal issues, along with identification of possible solutions for each problem listed. Some common problems
and potential solutions are outlined in Table 6-2. Because it is frequently impossible to address all medical and functional concerns with a wheelchair alone,
problem solving is characterized by the setting of priorities and compromise.
It may be necessary to identify alternative solutions to the problems identified
(eg, surgical, medical, therapeutic alternatives).

Provide a Stable Base

Sitting can be a stable position from which to perform functional ADL.
Stability begins at the base of support. A well-constructed wheelchair frame
and a firm seat and back can provide a good basis for stability. Naugahyde
upholstery, standard on most wheelchairs, does not provide the patient with
a stable base from which to function. Postural correction or accommodation
are not possible with standard upholstery. In fact, the "hammock" effect of
the sling seat and back actually can create postural problems (see Fig. 6-3) and
subsequent secondary problems (ie, pain, skin breakdown). The firm-based
seat and back, if fitted and prescribed individually, can effectively equalize
weight-bearing forces, correct flexible deformities, and support fixed
deformities.

Correct Flexible Deformities; Accommodate Fixed Deformities

Correction of flexible problems and accommodation of fixed deformities
is accomplished through the use of a variety of seating system components as
outlined in Table 6-2. It is important to provide proximal correction first, beginning with the pelvis, since proximal posture influences distal posture and
function. Failure to follow a proximal to distal direction for provision of seating
solutions may result in overtreatment of the problems.

Provide the Least Restrictive System Possible

Probably the most important principle of seating is the provision of maximal support with the least restrictive system possible. *It is crucial to allow
the patient to use any available motor control.* At the same time, available
energy should not be consumed in simply maintaining the upright position.
Removable parts, such as head or neck rests, can be used as the patient fatigues.
These accessories may significantly increase sitting tolerance.

Provide a Trial Period

Final decisions about the seating and mobility needs should be reserved
until the proposed solutions are tested. Trial systems can be easily and inexpensively built with triwall cardboard and various foams. Techniques of mock-

Table 6-2. Common Problems and Possible Solutions

Body Segment	Common Problems	Possible Solution(s)
Pelvis	Flexible posterior tilt	Firm seat and back with belt placed at an angle of 45° to sitting surface
		Lumbar roll or lumbar corset
	Fixed posterior tilt	Accommodate with semireclining backrest
	Flexible obliquity	Firm seat and back with belt placed at an angle of 45° to sitting surface
		Pelvic block pads to maintain midline position
	Fixed obliquity	Accommodate by building up seat or cushion under high side
Hips	Hip adduction	Proper pelvic position
		Abductor pommel placed at most distal point on seat midline (easily removable)
	Hip extension, flexible	Proper pelvic position
		Increase flexion past 90° with inclinable seat or wedge cushion
	Hip extension, fixed	Accommodate with reclining back wheelchair
Thigh	Thigh length discrepancy	Proper pelvic position
		Asymmetrical seat depth
Knees	Flexion contracture	Accommodate with shorter seat depth and footplates which extend posteriorly
		Proper pelvic position
	Extension contracture	Accommodate with elevating leg rests
Feet	Fixed deformities	Support with foot cradle
Spine	Poor trunk control; no asymmetries	Proper pelvic position
		Lateral supports mounted on high back
		Reclined back, inclined seat (maintain 90° seat-to-back angle)
	Fair trunk control; no asymmetries	Lateral supports used part-time especially in transit
	Flexible scoliosis	Proper pelvic position
		Three-point pressure system
	Fixed scoliosis	Proper pelvic position
		Three-point pressure system for support
		Total contact system may be indicated for skin protection
	Flexible kyphosis	Proper pelvic position
		Lumbar roll
		Clavicular pads
		Reclined back, inclined seat (maintain 90° seat-to-back angle)
	Fixed kyphosis	Accommodate with concave backrest or heavy padding
Shoulder girdle	Excessive protraction	Firm back
		Clavicular pads
	Excessive retraction	Concave backrest
		Lap tray
		Humeral wings on tray
Head and neck	Poor head control	Proper pelvic alignment
		Reclined back, inclined seat
		Posterolateral head rest
		Anterior restraint for car transport
		Cervical orthosis may be indicated
	Fair head control	Removable head rest—used especially for travel
	Goosenecking	Proper alignment of pelvis and spine

up fabrication are described in detail by Bergen and Colangelo,[12] and trial of possible solutions is approached in a proximal to distal direction. That is, one should start at the base of support and work up and out from there. The ideal position for postural alignment is the goal for each body segment. When that is not attainable, the goals are to equalize weight-bearing and optimize comfort and function. Input from the patient must be considered very seriously during the trial phase. A position that appears to be "therapeutically correct" may actually be uncomfortable to the patient. If fear or resistance to change is suspected, it may be helpful to introduce the new position gradually through several small modifications spread over time.

Provide Commercially Available Equipment

The equipment is ordered after final decisions are made about what components are needed. Whenever possible, commercially available solutions should be provided. Custom specifications should be limited in order to reduce costs and delivery time.[4] Commercially available options for meeting seating and mobility needs are improving almost daily. Manufacturers are responding to the demands created by requests from the growing number of knowledgeable clinicians. Equipment that once required custom design and construction can now be ordered as an accessory or option for the standard wheelchair. Custom design and construction essentially are needed only for the very severely disabled person with multiple fixed deformities. Most elderly patients, even those residing in nursing homes, can be fitted with commercially available equipment.

COMMON POSITIONING PROBLEMS

Most postural problems originate at the pelvis. When the pelvis is out of ideal alignment, weight-bearing distortion, discomfort, and increased risk of skin breakdown result. The two most common seating problems are posterior pelvic tilt and pelvic obliquity. The many ramifications of these postural problems and some possible solutions are discussed in detail.

Posterior Pelvic Tilt

Excessive posterior pelvic tilt in sitting is a common problem frequently seen even among the able-bodied. Sometimes referred to as "sacral sitting," this postural problem can originate from physical problems such as proximal weakness or extensor spasticity but more commonly results from insufficient support being provided by the seating surface. Gravity tends to pull the pelvis posteriorly in sitting (Fig. 6-2). This deviation will occur if the forces of gravity are not counteracted with muscle action or forces from the seat and back surfaces. Naugahyde upholstery does not provide enough support to counteract

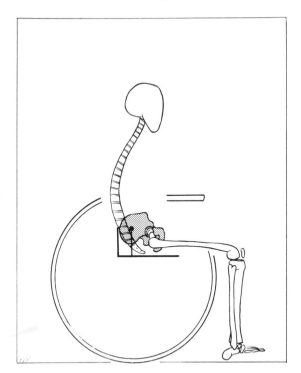

Fig. 6-2. Gravitational force pulls pelvis posteriorly into sacral sitting. Note resultant positions of hips and spine.

gravity; thus, the pelvis tilts posteriorly in the presence of weakness or paralysis.

The dangers of prolonged sitting in a posterior pelvic tilt are numerous. Biomechanically, the posterior pelvic tilt is consistent with a hip position of extension, adduction, and internal rotation, and a spinal posture of forward flexion. The position of the spine is a compensatory strategy to permit a forward vertical orientation for the head and the eyes (a righting response). This posture, illustrated in Figure 6-2, is in direct contrast to the ideal postural alignment previously described (Fig. 6-1).

The earliest symptom of posterior pelvic tilt is discomfort of the back, shoulders, or neck. If allowed to persist, worsening of the postural problem may result as the patient tries, ineffectively, to relieve discomfort. The most serious problem resulting from persistence of the posterior pelvic tilt is sacral skin breakdown. When the pelvis is tilted posteriorly, most of the weight-bearing forces are placed on the sacrum. Unlike the ischial tuberosities, which are well padded by the gluteals, the sacrum is covered only with a thin layer of skin. It simply is not designed for weight-bearing. Normal age-related changes in the skin are present for most elderly, increasing susceptibility to sacral ulcers.[1]

The best and easiest solution for the flexible posterior pelvic tilt is to provide a firm seat and back placed at an angle of 90° to each other. When combined with a pelvic belt placed at an angle of 45° from the seating surface, a three-point pressure system is created to counteract the effects of gravity. The direction of counteracting forces is illustrated in Figure 6-1. It is important that the belt be positioned just below the anterior superior iliac spines (ASIS) to anchor the pelvis back in the chair. If pressure is applied directly over the ASIS, the pelvis tends to tip posteriorly. This solution will only work, however, if the pelvis, back, and hips are flexible enough to achieve the ideal neutral positioning. (This will have been determined in the evaluation phase by assessment of flexibility and symmetry.)

Treatment of fixed postural problems requires a different strategy. Accommodation of the problem is provided to improve comfort and function and to equalize weight-bearing and minimize the risk of skin breakdown. Limited hip range of motion is accommodated by opening up of the seat-to-back angle by use of a reclining or semireclining back. Accommodation of lack of flexibility between the low back and the pelvis may require the addition of a well-padded or concave backrest to prevent excessive weight-bearing on the lumbar or thoracic spinous processes.

Pelvic Obliquity

Another common seating problem is pelvic obliquity. This is essentially a lateral tipping of the pelvis with one ischial tuberosity sitting higher than the other. This pelvic position is mechanically consistent with a compensatory scoliosis because of the natural tendency to right the head to a forward, vertical position. The hips assume an asymmetrical posture simply because they are attached to an asymmetrical pelvis.

As illustrated in Figure 6-3, the hammock effect of the standard sling seat and back wheelchair is commonly responsible for this postural problem. One side of the ischium sinks into the lowest point of the hammock, creating pelvic obliquity. Physical problems, including asymmetric muscle tone, asymmetric weakness, and pelvic fractures, may also cause or contribute to this problem.

The flexible pelvic obliquity is corrected in the same way as the posterior pelvic tilt—with a firm seat and back combined with a pelvic belt. A structural pelvic obliquity requires accommodation to equalize weight-bearing. The space between the seat and high side of the pelvic obliquity is filled by building up the seat surface (Fig. 6-4) with asymmetric density foams (soft foam on the low side, medium to dense foam on the high side). An alternative to foams is a dual-channel, air-filled cushion. The channel on the high side is filled with more air than the low side. In either case, the lower side continues to sit lower, but the high side will accept some of the weight-bearing forces. The identification of the correct combination of foams or air pressure to equalize weight-bearing is essentially a matter of trial and error. Measurement of weight-bearing equality can be accomplished subjectively if the examiner places hands, palms up, between the ischial tuberosities and seat surface. A pneumatic pressure gauge permits a more objective measurement.[13] This alternative, which is new to the commercial market, is still rather costly.

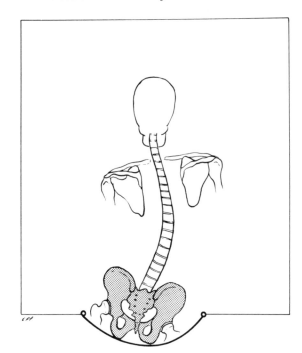

Fig. 6-3. Pelvic obliquity from hammock effect of sling-style seat. Note compensatory scoliosis.

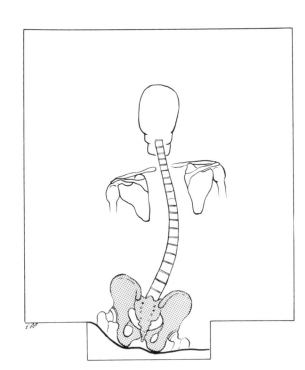

Fig. 6-4. Accommodation of fixed pelvic obliquity to equalize weight-bearing and reduce risk of skin breakdown.

Correction and Accommodation of Distal Problems

Treatment of postural problems at the pelvis will generally correct flexible, distal problems. If the more distal problems still exist once the pelvis is corrected or accommodated, correction or accommodation is provided as needed. The seat, back, and belt are the most commonly needed accessories for the standard wheelchair frame. Other accessories or modifications may include external supports to assist with positioning of the pelvis, lower extremities, trunk, neck or head, and/or feet. Table 6-2 lists common problems and potential solutions. *The basic principles apply to the solving of any seating problems; that is, one should always progress from proximal to distal body parts, strive for a functionally optimal position with neutral alignment, correct flexible deformities, and support fixed deformities.*

EQUIPMENT OPTIONS

Several firm seat and back systems are commercially available. Most are constructed from wood and foam and clip onto the wheelchair frame to allow folding and portability. Firm seats and backs need not be wood, however. Plastics and adjustable tension fabrics can provide the necessary forces to counteract the gravitational pull and add less weight to the chair. Stock residential wheelchairs can be "customized" easily by adding commercially available seat and back inserts over the naugahyde upholstery. It is important to mount the inserts in a way that prevents asymmetry caused when only one side of the insert rests on the wheelchair tubing. Inserts sized to fit between the tubing can usually be held in place with Velcro straps, whereas inserts cut to sit over the tubing generally must be attached with metal clip-on hardware. Alternatively one can add a wood or plastic base to the underside of the wheelchair cushion. Many cushion covers will accommodate the addition of a $\frac{1}{4}$- to $\frac{1}{2}$-in thick ABS plastic base. Care should be taken to round the corners of the plastic, however, to prevent punctures in the cushion cover.

The seating system would not be complete without a pressure-relieving cushion. The seat cushion provides comfort and increased sitting tolerance for the patient who has sensation and protection against excess pressures for the patient who has none. Little scientific data exists regarding the comparative effectiveness of various wheelchair cushions. There are, however, some parameters on which to base the decision for wheelchair cushion choice. Among other considerations are the weight of the patient, the patient's own feelings of security and comfort, finances, and individual problems, such as urinary incontinence and history of skin problems while using a particular type of cushion.

Foam cushions are generally the least expensive and can be quite effective in distributing weight-bearing forces. The life of foams are limited, however, and must be watched closely for wear and breakdown.[14] Foams conform best to body contours when covered with polyester or other elasticized fabric and are subject to damage from urinary incontinence. Gel-filled cushions are generally more expensive than foams but are urine resistant. One potential drawback to gel cushions is that they can be heavy and awkward to lift, making independent management difficult for the elderly. Air-filled cushions are becoming increasingly popular. They can be quite expensive but are effective and easy to clean. Potential disadvantages of air-filled cushions include difficulty of maintaining appropriate pressures[15] and the patient's feelings of instability while seated on the cushion.

Purchase of the most appropriate equipment requires familiarity with commercially available options. Maintenance of an up-to-date "library" of manufacturers' catalogs is essential. Wheelchair vendors and manufacturers generally will provide information without hesitation as well as in-service education on request. It is impossible to make knowledgeable recommendations about seating and mobility systems without up-to-date information.

CASE EXAMPLE

This case is presented to illustrate many of the seating and mobility problems discussed in this chapter. The patient was discharged from a rehabilitation unit to her home. However, many of the principles illustrated in this case apply to patients in other environments, including long-term care facilities.

Background Information

A. S. is a 68-year-old woman who 8 weeks ago had a right cerebrovascular accident (CVA). She is now medically stable and ready for discharge home where she lives with her 72-year-old retired husband. She will receive physical therapy services from the visiting nurses' association. The wheelchair evaluation revealed the following information.

Musculoskeletal Status

Range of motion (ROM) for A. S. is within functional limits. She has no structural problems that prevent good postural alignment in sitting. Several flexible deviations are noted when the patient is seated in her current wheelchair. The pelvis is tilted posteriorly and is rotated forward on the left side. The spine is generally kyphotic with a decrease in the lumbar lordosis, an increase in the thoracic kyphosis, and an increase in the cervical lordosis ("goosenecking"). All these deviations are eliminated when the patient is seated in a straight-backed chair with a pelvic positioning belt. There is evidence of left glenohumeral subluxation, which is being supported with a conventional hemiplegic sling. She complains of pain in the left shoulder which "seems to be there only during and after range of motion exercises" or if she "moves the wrong way in bed."

All patient measurements are symmetrical. Back of buttocks to back of knee, $17\frac{1}{2}$ in; back of knee to bottom of foot, 16 in; across hips, $12\frac{1}{2}$ in; seat height to axilla, 16 in.

Neuromuscular Status

Right upper and lower extremities are within normal limits. There is a flaccid paralysis of the left side with no evidence of tonic reflex activity or protective reactions.

Functional Status

The patient is able to walk short distances using a long leg brace on the left and a small-base quad cane. Walking distance is reportedly limited by claudication which was a problem even prior to the onset of the hemiplegia. She is expected to use the wheelchair as the main form of long distance travel and at least part of the time at home. It is probable that she will wear the long leg brace while sitting in the wheelchair. The patient transfers using a stand-pivot to the right, requiring minimal assistance and cueing for safety. This is assumed to be the technique that will be used at the time of discharge from the hospital. Once at home, the patient expects to resume some of her previous activities, including community travel with family and friends, who will be lifting the wheelchair in and out of cars. Some wheelchair-related functional problems were identified by the family: (1) the patient could not sit close to the dining room table in the current wheelchair; (2) she had difficulty ascending built-up thresholds in some of the rooms at home; and (3) plush carpet throughout the house made wheelchair propulsion difficult.

Current Wheelchair

The patient is presently seated in a standard adult-sized hemiplegic wheelchair which belongs to the hospital. It has a sling seat and back, solid rubber tires, and an elevating leg rest on the left. She is using a 3-in high-density foam cushion on the seat and a lumbar support pillow on the back to accommodate for the depth of the seat, which is too long for her. She is able to propel this wheelchair using her right upper and lower extremities but is limited because of difficulty in reaching the floor with her right foot. In addition, the back cushion has moved her forward from the rear wheel, making it difficult to achieve an efficient push on the rim. She is able to lock and unlock the brakes independently, using a brake extension on the left. Sitting posture is poor, secondary to the hammock effect of the sling seat and back. The pelvic position seems secondary to the seat depth (too long) and the placement of her left foot on the leg rest.

Identified Problems

1. The patient has poor sitting posture in current wheelchair, with increased trunk flexion, protraction of the shoulders, posterior tilting of the pelvis, left side of pelvis rotated forward in relation to the right;

2. The standard seat depth is too long, and accommodation with back cushion creates a disadvantage for the right upper extremity in propelling the wheelchair;

3. The seat height of the present chair is too high for optimal use of right lower extremity for propulsion;

4. The patient requires lightweight chair to allow for lifting in/out of car;

5. The patient requires full-length armrests to assist in stand-pivot transfer but these make it difficult for the patient to have meals while sitting in the wheelchair;

6. The patient has difficulty propelling the wheelchair over carpeting and small obstacles (thresholds).

Recommended Solutions

1. A lightweight hemiplegic wheelchair frame is recommended to allow low seat position and relative ease of lifting the chair in and out of the car.

2. A wood and foam (2-in high-density foam) seat (14 in wide × 16 in deep) and back (14 in wide × 16 in high) to improve stability and posture, to equalize weight-bearing forces and to protect the integrity of the skin while the patient is seated in the wheelchair.

3. A Velcro-close pelvic belt, mounted at an angle of 45° to the seat and back to hold the pelvis back in the chair in a symmetrical posture.

4. Clip-on hardware to be mounted on seat and back to allow for easy removal when the chair is lifted in and out of the car. Seat hardware should be bent to achieve the lowest possible seat height (seat level with horizontal tubing) to increase ease of propulsion.

5. Pneumatic tires and semipneumatic casters to increase the ease of propulsion outdoors, over small obstacles, and carpets.

6. A quick-release mechanism for the rear wheels to allow for removal for lifting wheelchair in and out of the car.

7. Anti-tipping devices for safety.

8. Removable, adjustable-height, full-length armrests to aid with stand-pivot transfer; these can be removed or lowered so that the patient can sit at a table or desk.

9. Brake extensions.

10. Footrests with oversized footplates that extend backward to allow

for closer to 90° angle at the left knee, reducing the tendency for forward rotation of the pelvis on the left side.

11. Cane and crutch holder to allow the patient to carry the quad cane on the back of the chair.

Trial Period

Trial of proposed seating changes was accomplished with a cardboard and foam mock-up built onto the hospital chair. The patient had no difficulty tolerating the new system, and improvements in posture and function were noticed immediately. The wheelchair was ordered as recommended. All components were commercially available.

SUMMARY

The need for a wheelchair prescription may be brought about by various illnesses or disorders that commonly occur in the elderly patient, including stroke, lower extremity amputation, spinal cord injury, multiple sclerosis, Parkinson's disease, and many others. Individualized assessment of wheelchair needs is the mechanism through which independent function and comfort can be maximized, while risk of secondary disability is minimized.

The cost of individualized wheelchair prescription need not be prohibitive. A stock institutional chair can be adapted rather inexpensively with seat and back inserts and relocation of safety belts to act as pelvic-positioning aids. If more extensive modification is needed, however, justification of cost is not difficult. *One must compare the cost of an appropriate wheelchair to the cost of treating secondary disabilities that may result from the use of an inappropriate wheelchair.* Costs incurred while a decubitus ulcer or other secondary disability heals easily exceed wheelchair modification costs.

REFERENCES

1. Itoh M, Lee, MHM: Rehabilitation for the aged. p. 1. In Jackson O (ed): Physical Therapy of the Geriatric Patient, Churchill Livingstone, New York, 1983
2. Gans BM, Hallenborg SC: Wheelchair prescription for the physically disabled. In Positioning: Maximizing Form for Maximum Function. Everest & Jennings, Camarillo, California, 1984
3. Gans BM, Hallenborg SC: Power-driven wheelchairs: Making the right choices. Rx Home Care :32, 1984
4. Lobley S, Freed MM, Dutton N, Smith R: Wheelchair prescription and design for the individual with neurologic impairment. Semin Neurol 3:171, 1983
5. Hartigan J: The dangerous wheelchair. J Am Geriatr Soc 30:572, 1982
6. Daniels L, Worthingham C: Muscle Testing. 4th Ed. WB Saunders, Philadelphia, 1980

7. Capute AJ, Accardo PJ: Primitive Reflex Profile. University Park Press, Baltimore, 1978

8. Hoskins TA, Squires JE: Developmental assessments: a test for gross motor and reflex development. In Determining Abilities of Children with Central Nervous System Disorders. American Physical Therapy Association, Washington, D.C., 1975

9. Jackson O, Lang RH: Functional evaluation of the elderly. p. 203. In Jackson O (ed): Physical Therapy of the Geriatric Patient. Churchill Livingstone, New York, 1983

10. Shinnar SE: Use of adaptive equipment in feeding the elderly. J Am Diet Assoc 83:321, 1983

11. Solomon K: Psychosocial dysfunctions in the aged: Assessment and intervention. In Jackson O (ed):Physical Therapy of the Geriatric Patient. Churchill Livingstone, New York, 1983

12. Bergen A, Colangelo C: Positioning the Client With Central Nervous System Deficits: The Wheelchair and Other Adapted Equipment. Valhalla Rehabilitation Publications, Valhalla, New York, 1982

13. Garber SL, Krouskop TA, Carter RE: A system for clinically evaluating wheelchair pressure relief cushions. Am J Occup Ther 32:565, 1978

14. Noble PC, Goode BL, Krouskop TA, Crisp B: The response of polyurethane foam wheelchair cushions to environmental aging. p. 218. In Proceedings of the 6th Annual Conference on Rehabilitation Engineering, 1983

15. Williams R, Krouskop T, Noble P, Brown J: The influence of inflation pressure on the effectiveness of air-filled wheelchair cushions. p. 215. In Proceedings of the 6th Annual Conference on Rehabilitation Engineering, 1983

7 | Gait Characteristics

Jacquelin Perry

Walking is an activity that uses the lower extremities to carry the body from one location to another. The limbs repetitiously perform a set of motions which simultaneously maintain a stable upright posture while also providing forward progression.

Normal function depends on (1) free passive joint mobility, (2) appropriate timing of muscle action, and (3) appropriate intensity of muscle action. The major physiological factors are connective tissue flexibility, muscle strength, and selective neural control.[1] The basic physiological requirements must be met by each joint involved in walking. The demands placed on the body during walking are bilaterally equal.

Aging can lead to several physical changes: (1) Muscle strength is reduced; (2) reaction times are slowed; (3) connective tissue stiffens; and (4) bones are less dense and more vulnerable to fracture.

Another possible effect of aging is the increased opportunity to experience injury or illness and consequently acquire residual disability.[2-4] Osteoarthritis is a good example. Because the mechanism is a deficit in the natural repair process of cartilage, the pathology accumulates with age. Its occurrence, however, is cause-related rather than a spontaneous event. Abnormal joint stresses are introduced by malformations following trauma, infection, developmental errors (postural distortions), or faulty metabolism.[4a] The latter may relate to a genetic predisposition in some populations, such as the English.[5] Inconsistency in the timing and location of pathology and improved diagnostic capability contradict the earlier assumption that degenerative joint changes are a natural aging event. Similarly, the neurological causes of impaired walking ability in the elderly person are more frequently related to specific pathologies which can also be found in other age groups.[6-10] Hence, normal aging is not a primary cause of walking disturbances in the elderly.

There are thus two elderly populations: healthy individuals experiencing normal aging, and persons who have acquired subtle forms of physical im-

113

pairment. Normally aged persons are free of symptoms, clinical signs, and medications. This is not true for those who have residual pathology.

In the following review of the effects of aging on a person's ability to walk, healthy subjects are differentiated from those with subtle degrees of physical impairment. For an example of the impaired elderly, data from an ambulatory group of patients with joint pain who volunteered for a rehabilitation activity program are used.

MEASUREMENTS OF FUNCTION

The quality of a person's ambulatory performance generally is judged by the pattern of motion displayed at the individual joints. One looks for smoothness as well as appropriateness of the arc of movement.[11] Motion is easy to observe or capture on film but difficult to translate into quantitated values, which limits the data available. Alternatively, one can measure the effectiveness of a person's gait pattern by noting the individual stride characteristics: (1) the speed of travel, (2) the stride length, and (3) the energy cost of walking. All three gait parameters are considered in this study of the effects of aging.

Joint Motion—Alterations With Aging

Range of motion (ROM) studies have failed to identify significant differences between healthy subjects >60 years of age as compared with younger adults 20 to 40 years of age.[12,13] This degree of "normalcy" is reflected in their gait measurements. Only two minor differences were found in a study of healthy elderly subjects (60 to 65 years of age) compared with similar groups in each younger decade, from the second decade to the fifth.[13] First, the arc of passive plantar flexion occurring in preswing was ~5° less for the elderly than the 20° displayed by the younger subjects. All age groups used an equal amount of dorsiflexion (10°) in the preceding terminal stance phase. The difference, most probably, is an indirect indication of reduced triceps surae muscle force. Weaker muscles have less tissue turgor and thus less rebound when released. Second, at the hip, the older subjects exhibited slightly more flexion (35 vs 30°). Their hip extension of 10° equaled that of the other ages.

No differences in knee function were found. The common pattern was 20° of knee flexion during limb loading, full extension in terminal stance, and 70° flexion in initial swing.

A subsequent study of the joint motions used during walking included men 67 through 87 years of age. The elderly group showed small but consistent decreases (5°) in most arcs of motion that were most consistent for men in their seventies or eighties. Similar differences were exhibited by 70-year-old women.[14]

Thus, while aging may lead to slight stiffening of the connective tissues, the changes are not sufficient to alter the walking pattern of the healthy aged.

This is logical because the maximum arcs of motion used in walking represent only one-half of the normal range of knee flexion and ankle plantar and one-third of normal hip flexion. Motion in the opposite directions was similarly unchallenged. Hence, there is a large functional margin to accommodate minor tissue changes. These findings indicate that continued activity maintains connective tissue health and hence its free mobility. The reports of water loss and chemical change associated with aging are the same as those found in immobilization studies.[15] Hence, the changes may relate not to age per se, but indicate instead the level of activity of one's lifestyle.

Stride Characteristics

Effectiveness of a person's walking pattern is indicated by several stride characteristics. Each characteristic presented represents a different facet in the walking complex (gait velocity, stride length, and cadence).

Gait Velocity

Gait velocity is the composite measure.[16] It represents the distance (meters) one can walk in a set time (minute). Among different studies, average values for normal adult function ranged from 77.4 to 87.0 m/min.[13,14,16,17] Healthy aging caused only minor slowing. A group of 20 nonimpaired elderly, 60 to 87 years of age, had a walking speed of 78.6 m/min.[19] This is 5 percent less than the mean for 140 persons <60 years of age (82.6 m/min, average 31 years) tested in the same laboratory. The difference, however, falls within 1 SD (10.6 m/min) of the younger group's average velocity.[19] It is also similar to the normal velocity of 77.4 m/min reported by Findley who covertly observed people walking in various areas in the community.[14] Direct comparisons of average gait velocities for elderly and young groups consistently show slowing with age.[13] Findley[14] found a 14 percent decrease in walking speed for persons averaging 74 years of age as compared with young adults 30 years of age. Most of his elderly subjects had some degree of arthritis and used multiple medications. An analysis of slow, usual, and fast walking also showed that the elderly (67 years of age) were relatively slower than the young group (25 years of age) at each effort level.[20] The difference was 11 percent for the usual and fast paces and 22 percent at the slow pace. All elderly subjects had been carefully screened for signs or symptoms of disability.

Greater change was found in the group of impaired elderly subjects undergoing rehabilitation for joint pain.[20a] Their average gait velocity of 64 m/min was a 19 percent reduction from the normal standard.[10] By making the extra effort to walk rapidly, these subjects reached but did not exceed the normal free velocity of 83 m/min. Persons with confirmed degenerative hip disease registered a range of walking speeds from 10 to 80 percent of normal (mean 45 percent N). Their walking ability following total hip arthroplasty averaged 75 percent of normal.[10]

It is clinically significant when setting gait standards for elderly persons to be careful to differentiate between normal healthy aging and the sequelae of acquired disability. *Aging per se introduces an ~10 percent slowing in average walking speed.* This difference, however, falls within the broad range of "normal" registered by different laboratories. Changes from pathology will vary with the severity of the physical impairment.

Stride Length and Cadence

Stride length and cadence are the basic determinants of a person's gait velocity. Of the two, stride length is the stronger factor. It averages 1.5 m in normal subjects.[17] The healthy elderly had a slightly shorter stride of 1.39 m, a 7 percent reduction.[18] Murray et al found a 15 percent difference, and Findley's elderly group evidenced a 19 percent decrease.[14] The elderly group with joint pain had a significantly shorter stride of 1.18 m, 21 percent less than normal performance. Even during their fast effort, these impaired elderly subjects could only increase their stride 11 percent to 1.31 m. Murray found no age influence on stride width. The major determinant of stride length is the arc of hip motion, which is very evident in patients with a painful hip.

Cadence (or step rate) is a less significant component of gait velocity because it is more easily altered voluntarily.[21] Generally, stride length and cadence are reduced proportionally. Many patients who still have sufficient strength or who are not in too much pain increase their step rate to reduce the effects of a shortened stride. In this way, there is less loss of walking speed. The normal cadence value is 112 steps per minute. A nonsignificant increase to 114 was registered by the healthy elderly. Findley's elderly subjects also partially compensated for their shortened stride length by an increased step rate of 4 percent.[14] The impaired elderly had a slower cadence of 107. In their effort to walk fast, step rate was increased 20 percent (129 steps/min) whereas the gain in stride length was only 11 percent.

Single Limb Support

Single limb support is a major factor in stride length because it reflects both body balance and weight tolerance of the limb. The latter is strongly influenced by muscle strength and pain. Normally, each limb spends 40 percent of the gait cycle in the single-support phase. This occurred in the healthy elderly. Those with joint pain exhibited a minor reduction to 38 percent of the gait cycle. Patients with diagnosed osteoarthritis of the hip had major reductions in single-limb-support times.

Foot Support Pattern

The foot support pattern showed two age variations relating to heel rise. Peak elevation of the heel was 6 percent less for the subjects >74 years of age, and it occurred later. Both changes are consistent with decreased calf muscle strength. The decrease in hip extension at the end of the single-stance period is another contributor to these changes in the foot support pattern. A delay in heel rise during terminal stance also has been found to correlate with the person's general activity level.

Thus, healthy elderly persons, even in the age range between 70 and 80 years, exhibited only minor motion changes. There was a reduction in gait velocity, stride length, and heel rise. With normal passive joint mobility and no aberrant motion occurring to indicate impaired neural control, the primary cause must be decreased muscle strength.

MUSCLE WEAKNESS RELATIONSHIPS TO GAIT CHARACTERISTICS

Regardless of age, a person must accomplish three basic tasks in walking; weight acceptance, single-limb support, and limb advancement. In meeting these requirements as well as in providing transitional preparations for stance and swing, eight distinct patterns of motion and muscle action are performed. Adequate muscle force to restrain the effects of gravity during stance and to advance the limb quickly in swing is essential. Limitation resulting from muscle weakness is evidenced by a gait error or slowness of action.

Muscle strength is most commonly assessed by manual testing, using the international five-point scale (0 to 5). It is assumed that the numerical and strength differences are equivalent. Significant discrepancies between test results and patient function have occurred with this system. This area of confusion has been clarified by quantitated interpretations of the manual muscle test. Grade 5 (normal) strength in patients who have had polio proved to be only 75 percent of true normal.[22] Similarly, the quadriceps muscle of patients with a patellectomy, which was graded normal by manual testing, had only 60 percent of the strength registered by the other limb.[8] The finding that grade 4 (good) in the polio patients was 40 percent of true normal has been anatomically confirmed by anterior horn cell counts.[23] Grade 3 (fair) averaged 15 percent. Hence, although the manual strength test is most convenient, the finding must be reinterpreted. Manual muscle testing also presumes normal skeletal alignment in the position used for testing.

The functional demands presented to the muscles are more easily appreciated when expressed as a percentage of the person's maximum isometric strength and when quantitated values are used. Normal adult strength varies markedly with the person's vocational and athletic habits. For representative values, one must assess a population that mixes recreational sports and a sedentary occupation. Conveniently, this is the group most available for testing.

The effects of aging can be gained from three critical muscles that have been measured in both the young and elderly. These are the hip abductors, knee extensors, and ankle plantar flexors. Reported normal male hip abductor strength ranged between 11.2[24] and 13.9 kg[25] for an average of 12.6 kg. The women averaged 35 percent less. Strength values for quadriceps varied between 12[26,27] and 26 kg[28,29] for an average of 18.8 kg for men; again the women's values were 30 percent less. Equivalent measurements for a group of healthy elderly persons showed no loss of hip abductor strength, but the quadriceps' values were 28 percent weaker. The impaired elderly group showed 33 percent loss of abductor strength and 47 percent loss of quadriceps strength.

Both elderly populations showed the greatest strength loss in the ankle plantar flexors. Normal male strength averaged 15 kg[30]; the women were 54 percent weaker. Among the elderly subjects, plantar flexor strength was virtually equal for men and women (5.2 and 5.5 kg, respectively). Hence, a proportionally greater loss was found in the men, 66 percent as compared to 21 percent. Plantar flexor strength for the impaired aged population was reduced in an additional 20 percent. Despite these significant reductions in strength, manual testing would have graded them as normal. The force an examiner can exert against the supine patient's foot is <15 kg, a challenge far less than body weight. Testing of the subject's standing was more informative. Most of the disabled elderly displayed their limitation by a reduction in the height and number of heel rises they could accomplish.

The significance of these decreases in available strength can be realized best by reviewing the muscle demands occurring in the average gait cycle. During walking the most vigorous muscle action is required in stance as the downward accelerations of body weight are restrained.[30a] There are four significant groups; hip extensors and abductors, quadriceps, and ankle plantar flexors. Each has a specific task that must be repeated with every stride. Thus, two factors are involved: absolute strength to counter the force of dropping body weight and endurance to perform this task an indefinite number of times. Faster gait velocities reduce the duration of the muscles' actions but increase the instantaneous force required. Conversely, muscle weakness necessitates reducing the force demands by using a slower velocity. Endurance will be compromised by the longer time required to travel the desired distance. Resistance to the effects of aging by the endurance-rich type 1 muscle fibers preserves more function than one would expect from direct strength measurements. This physiological bias, however, does not fully compensate for the gross strength loss. The optimum compromise between muscle capability and functional demand is reflected by the person's spontaneous stride characteristics and motion pattern.

Weight Acceptance

Weight acceptance is the period of greatest demand. It involves two phases of motion—initial contact and loading. To preserve standing stability, the hip and knee extensor and hip abductor muscles must respond promptly in a coordinated manner. At initial floor contact, the flexed posture of the hip (30°) combined with residual forward momentum creates a need for extensor muscle action to stabilize both the trunk and limb. As body weight drops onto the limb, normal gluteus maximus and adductor magnus response is 30 percent of maximum strength.[19] Activity at this intensity is brief because the demand is quickly reduced passively as progression continues. If the pelvis drops (anterior tilt) giving the muscle fibers a more favorable length, weaker hip muscles can meet the demand. Accompanying lordosis avoids increasing postural demand. Waters et al,[31] found hip extensor muscle strength at 15° flexion to be 41 percent greater than that available with the hip in full extension. Perhaps this advantage contributes to the slight flexion contracture that is common in the elderly.

Knee extensor muscle demands are potentially high but are minimized by the size of the quadriceps. Advancement of the tibia by the heel rocker during limb loading develops a flexion torque at the knee. The resulting motion acts as a shock absorber. Peak knee flexion of 15° occurs just as single limb support begins. In the young adult, this is restrained by the quadriceps contracting at 15 percent of maximum strength. Elderly persons (healthy and impaired) exert 20 and 28 percent of their available strength. Normally, further demands are rapidly reduced as the calf muscles begin their task of restraining tibial advancement. This provides a stable base over which the knee can extend progressively. As body weight moves ahead of the knee joint axis, the need for quadriceps action ceases.

Three substitutions are commonly used to decrease the quadriceps demand during the loading response. All are seen in elderly persons who have functional problems in ambulation. Initial contact is made with a lower foot position as a result of ankle plantar flexion (5 to 10°) and the knee being slightly flexed. Both actions reduce the heel lever that initiates knee flexion. A shortened stride lessens the rate of floor contact and thus the knee flexing force. Forward lean of the trunk (noted by Murray as increased hip flexion)[13] reduces the flexor torque by moving the body weight line closer to the knee axis.

Single Limb Support

Single limb support presents a three-dimensional challenge. Forward progression must continue while the entire body weight is on one limb. In addition, the center of the mass is medial to the area of support.

Lifting the opposite limb for swing removes a major source of balance. The trunk will fall to the unsupported side unless there is a rapid response by the hip abductor muscles to stabilize the pelvis. Indeed, to meet this demand, these muscles become active as the stance limb is first loaded. The initial response of the gluteus medius and minimus muscles is at 30 percent of the maximum level, catching the falling pelvis and restoring level alignment. The muscles then maintain balance by a lower intensity of action throughout the single stance period. *Preservation of normal abductor muscle strength by the healthy elderly indicates that pelvic stability is a basic function that does not vary with age. The 33 percent loss of strength evidenced by the elderly subjects with joint pain necessitates postural substitutions.* Shifting the trunk toward the stance limb to reduce the demand on the weak uncoordinated abductor muscles is the most efficient means of maintaining balance. If strength loss is bilateral, the trunk moves from side to side with each step, adding a waddling quality to the person's gait. Elderly persons with less postural control use a wider step. This serves to catch the falling trunk. They also shorten their swing phase to lessen the demand. The stride length is correspondingly reduced.

To preserve stance stability while permitting continued progression, the calf muscles are the critical source of limb control. Throughout midstance, they contract at a moderate level (20 percent of maximum) to restrain the rate of tibial advancement over the flat foot. The muscles yield as they stabilize so that the ankle can dorsiflex 10°. The intensity of action must then more than double in terminal stance to support body weight on the forefoot as the heel rises. Their normal period of action, thus, is lengthy (40 percent of the gait cycle) and vigorous.

Loss of calf muscle strength was the greatest change seen in both healthy and impaired elderly subjects. This may represent either chronic strain or subtle underutilization to reduce the limb-loading forces. Using the forefoot rocker to roll the body ahead of the area of support during terminal stance is the major contribution to forward propulsion. This, however, places the body into a free fall which must be stopped by the weight-accepting limb. Delay and/or reduction of heel rise proportionally lessens the body's forward fall. The ultimate caution is that there be no heel rise during single limb support. Although these adaptations of foot and ankle action reduce strength demands and facilitate balance, they also decrease stride length and gait velocity.

Intrinsic foot stability is a commonly overlooked concern. Loading the heel creates an eversion thrust at the subtalar joint. Then inversion is introduced as weight is transferred to the forefoot. Soleus control of the heel supplements subtalar stabilization by the tibialis posterior and the peroneals. Muscle weakness generally leads to a flattened arch and foot strain. A reduction of single stance time is the functional result of the changes in both ankle and foot control.

Limb Advancement

Although characterized as a swing-phase task, advancing the limb is also influenced by actions occurring in late stance. The carryover relates to the ease of having the foot clear the floor in initial swing. Once this task is accomplished, advancing the limb is not difficult.

PRESWING POSTURING

The normal heel rise that occurs in terminal stance limits the areas of support to the forefoot. Continued advancement of body weight across the metatarsal heads during the subsequent preswing phase increases tibial instability, and the knee passively flexes 40°. Then, as the hip flexor muscles carry the thigh forward in initial swing, the additional 20° of knee flexion needed for the foot to clear the ground follows with minimal local muscle action.

Without preswing posturing, however, the person must make a deliberate knee flexion effort. If this is insufficient, a toe drag and possible tripping will result. This pattern of dysfunction is consistent with the gait characteristics of 80-year-old patients hospitalized because of falling. Step length (22 cm) was very short, only 58 percent of that accomplished by other patients of the same age who were hospitalized for another reason. Gait velocity was correspondingly slow (0.2 m/s). Both the short steps and slow walking speed are consistent with weak calf muscles that deny the person a terminal stance heel rise. Persistent quadriceps stabilization of the knee occurs to counteract the tibial instability caused by calf muscle weakness. Hence, two subtle patterns of muscle dysfunction are likely to deny the elderly person adequate preswing knee posturing.

ENERGY COST

Muscular action uses energy. Although the instantaneous energizing process is anaerobic, oxygen is necessary for continued activity and provides a convenient means of measuring the amount of energy that walking requires.

Normal young adults average 13 ml O_2/kg/min when walking at their customary velocity (82 m/min). Proportionally more energy is required at faster velocities and less is required in slower walking. The healthy elderly subjects reflected this relationship in their rate of energy expenditure. They used 12.5 m O_2/kg/min for a velocity of 77 m/min. Both groups had an efficiency of 6.25 m/ml O_2/kg. Normal efficiency, however, was not exhibited by the painful elderly group. Their energy rate was similar (12.3 ml O_2/kg/min), yet their gait velocity was only 64 m/min, resulting in 5.2 m/ml O_2/kg. The slightly lower rate of oxygen use by the painful elderly (11.4 vs 12.5 ml O_2/kg/min) also suggested some deconditioning of the energy production system.

Hence, these patients' weakened muscles had to exert extra effort as subtle protective postures were used to reduce the stress on their painful joints. This reflects the potential for a progressive loss of function as the additional exertion becomes too costly in expenditure of energy. The ability to provide sufficient energy is another factor. The cardiopulmonary system delivers oxygen to the tissues. Reduced capability can result from decreased activity or physical impairment of the heart, lungs, or vessels. The slower gait velocity of the painful elderly group was a way of accommodating this added impairment but introduces another penalty: *that is, increased energy cost for the distance walked.* The normal standard for energy cost is 0.16 ml O_2/kg/m. This was also the net energy cost for the healthy elderly groups, whereas those with pain expended 0.23 ml O_2/kg for each meter traveled.

SUMMARY

Peak walking ability is exhibited by adults between the ages of 20 and 40 years. Elderly persons <73 years of age who remain healthy walk at a comparable rate and level of energy expenditure. Their velocity and stride length, however, tend to be at the lower margin of normal. Age also allows many people to acquire subtle forms of physical impairment as well as years. These people will have significant reductions in their walking rates and efficiency. Persons 75 to >80 years of age exhibited more consistent patterns of slowing, but total freedom from acquired impairment was not defined. Hence, one must conclude that age alone does not significantly decrease walking capability. Thus, when normal performance is lacking, therapists must look for signs of physical impairment and seek means of correcting them.

REFERENCES

1. Perry J: Integrated function of the lower extremity including gait analysis. p. 1161. In Cruess RL, Rennie WRJ (eds): Adult Orthopedics, Churchill Livingstone, New York, 1984
2. Bienenstock H, Fernando KR: Arthritis in the elderly. Med Clin North Am 60:1173, 1976
3. Ceder L, Ekelund L, Inerot S, et al: Rehabilitation after hip fractures in the elderly. Acta Orthop Scand 50:681, 1979
4. Steinberg FU: Gait disorders in old age. Geriatrics 21:134, 1966
4a. Andriola DJ: When an elderly patient complains of weakness. Geriatrics 33:79, 1978
5. Mankin HJ: The articular cartilages, cartilage healing and osteoarthritis. p. 163. In Cruess RL, Rennie WRJ (eds): Adult Orthopedics. Churchill Livingstone, New York, 1984
6. Barron RE: Disorders of gait related to the aging nervous system. Geriatrics 22:13, 1967
7. Beasley BA, Ford DH: Aging and the extrapyramidal system. Med Clin North Am 60:1315, 1976
8. Fisher CH: Hydrocephalus as a cause of disturbances of gait in the elderly. Neurology 32:1358, 1982
9. Guimaraes RM, Issacs B: Characteristics of the gait in old people who fall. Int J Rehab Med 2:177, 1980
10. Perry J, Antonelli D, Gronley JK, Greenberg R: Quantitated function correlated with physical impairment. National Institutes of Health report, Grant No. AM-1743L, 1980
11. Cunningham DA, Rechnitzer PA, Pearch ME, Donner AP: Determinants of self-selected walking pace across ages 19 to 66. J Gerontol 37:560, 1982
12. Murray MP: Gait as a total pattern of movement. Am J Phys Med 46:290, 1967
13. Murray MP, Kory RC, Clarkson BH: Walking patterns in healthy old men. J Gerontol 24:169, 1969
14. Findley FR, Cody KA, Finizie RV: Locomotion patterns in elderly women. Arch Phys Med Rehabil 50:140, 1967
15. Akeson WH, Amiel D, LaViolette D: The connective tissue response to immobility: an accelerated aging response? Exp Gerontol 3:289, 1968

16. Andriacchi TP, Ogle JA, Galante JO: Walking speed as a basis of normal and abnormal gait measurements. J Biomech 10:261, 1977

17. Waters RL, Perry J, Hislop HJ: Energetics: Application to the study and management of locomotor disability. Orthop Clin North Am 9:351, 1978

18. Perry J, Carter CC, Mortimore MA, Hislop HH: Lower extremity strength, energy cost and stride characteristics of walking of normal adults over age 60. (submitted for publication)

19. O'Brien M, Power K, Sanford S, et al: Temporal gait patterns in healthy young and elderly females. Physiother Can 35:323, 1983

20. Croninshield RD, Brand RA, Johnston RC: The effects of walking velocity and age on hip kinematics and kinetics. Clin Orthop 132:140, 1978

20a. Perry J, Greenberg R, Bechtel R: Comparative effectiveness of outpatient rehabilitation programs for elderly persons with joint pain. Gerontology Rehabilitation Center Report. NIHR, Department of Education grant no. G0088000800.

21. Beasley WC: Quantitative muscle testing, principles and application to research and clinical services. Arch Phys Med Rehabil 42:398, 1961

22. Sharrad WJW: Correlation between changes in the spinal cord and muscle paralysis in poliomyelitis. Proc R Soc Med 40:540, 1953

23. Inman VT: Functional aspects of the abductor muscles of the hip. J Bone Joint Surg 29:607, 1947

24. Murray MP, Sepic SB: Maximum isometric torque of hip abductor and adductor muscles. Phys Ther 48:1327, 1968

25. Lieb FJ, Perry J: Quadriceps function, an electromyographic study under isometric conditions. J Bone Joint Surg 53A:749, 1971

26. Smidt GL: Biomechanical analysis of knee flexion and extension. J Biomech 6:97, 1973

27. Hill JA, Moynes DR, Yocum LA, et al: Gait and functional analysis of patients following patellectomy. Orthopedics 6:724, 1983

28. Lindahl O, Movin A, Ringqvist I: Knee extension measurement of isometric force in different positions of the knee-joint. Acta Orthop Scand 40:79, 1969

29. La Tourette G, Perry J, Moore TM, Harvey JP: Fractures and dislocation of the tarsometatarsal joint. p.40. In Bateman JE, Trott AW (eds): The Foot and Ankle. Decker, Thieme-Stratton, New York, 1980

30. Waters RL, Perry J, McDaniels JM: The relative strength of the hamstrings during hip extension. J Bone Joint Surg 56A:1592, 1974

31. Lyons K, Peryr J, Gronley JK, et al: Timing and relative intensity of hip extensor and abductor muscles action during level and stair ambulation (an EMG study). Phys Ther 63:1597, 1983

8 | Acute Emergency Care

Jane St. Clair
Walter F. Pizzi
Dana Gage

Physical therapists working with elderly patients may find themselves practicing in a variety of settings. The shortening of lengths of stay in hospitals, combined with the emphasis in medicine on exercise testing and training of healthy individuals as well as individuals with heart disease or those at high risk for its development, have increased the need for physical therapy to be performed outside of the traditional hospital setting. These settings may include long-term care facilities, special housing for the elderly, or private homes. These trends serve to emphasize the need for the physical therapist to be trained in emergency medical care and, in some states, such training may be a legal requirement for licensing.

In a medical emergency, the physical therapist needs certain basic information about the patient and some basic training in basic life support/cardiopulmonary resuscitation.

The most important patient information is:

1. *Patient's medical diagnosis/diagnoses.* This is helpful in anticipating and/or recognizing common complications of the disease. For example, in a patient with heart disease, vigorous therapy may precipitate angina. In a diabetic patient, the onset of physical therapy may lead to a decrease in insulin needs, precipitating a tendency to hypoglycemia.

It is important to maintain good communication with the patient's primary physician and caretaker/family. The physician's telephone number should be readily accessible for each patient.

2. *Patient's medications and their side effects.* It is also important to be aware of how the patient uses medication for specific problems. For example, does a patient with angina take nitroglycerin? Where is it kept and does it

usually resolve the patient's anginal attack? Does a patient with asthma respond to use of an aerosol inhaler or require hospital treatment? Open communication with the patient helps establish guidelines for medication use both as a basis in developing the treatment program and during an emergency situation.

3. *Relationship of patient's illness to family/staff members.* How are complications usually managed? Does someone bring the patient nitroglycerin or is it kept in the patient's pocket or in the bathroom? Is someone in the family familiar with how the patient responds to the medication?

4. *Familiarity with accessing medical intervention.* In a nursing home or hospital, medical intervention may be accessed simply by ringing a call button; in a private setting, it may be necessary to alert a family member or to call an ambulance (in many cities, this is as simple as dialing 911). Check and be familiar with the local access number.

Once a determination is made that an emergency exists and help has been called, it may be necessary to administer basic life support/cardiopulmonary resuscitation until professional help arrives. Although these skills may never have to be used, both therapist and patient will feel more confident if the therapist is familiar with these lifesaving techniques. (First aid techniques are also useful.)

Certification in basic life support/cardiopulmonary resuscitation is renewed yearly. Classes in local areas are available through the American Heart Association or American Red Cross. Failure to maintain certification may leave the therapist legally liable.

The goal of this chapter is to sensitize the physical therapists to emergency medical problems frequently encountered in their work with elderly patients to serve as a springboard to seeking appropriate practical training.

It is also important to realize that patients have their own perception of their illness. Understanding the patient's perception is an important part of working with the patient and of maintaining open communication and an effective working partnership.

This chapter reviews the general principles of emergency response available to a physical therapist and includes special considerations for the elderly patient.

HIGH-RISK PATIENTS

The elderly patient is, as a natural part of the aging process, more susceptible to heart attack, stroke, congestive heart failure, and high blood pressure. Other factors that place the patient at greater risk of developing cardiovascular disease include: family history of heart disease, high blood pressure, cigarette smoking, high levels of cholesterol in the blood, diabetes, race (black), and gender (male). Lack of exercise, overweight, and stressful life style may also contribute to a patient's chances of having a heart attack.

Cardiovascular diseases cause more deaths in the United States each year than do all forms of cancer and other diseases combined. High blood pressure, atherosclerosis, heart attack, stroke, and congestive heart failure are forms of cardiovascular disease. High blood pressure (hypertension) can lead to stroke, heart attack, and kidney failure, and is a major risk factor of cardiovascular disease. Most people with high blood pressure have no symptoms at all. There are no specific warning signs, *especially among the elderly,* although persistent headaches, dizziness, fatigue, and tension sometimes occur with high blood pressure. The only accurate way to determine whether a patient has high blood pressure is to check blood pressure regularly. An adult with a systolic blood pressure of ≥140 mmHg or a diastolic blood pressure of ≥90 mmHg (at rest either sitting or lying down) at first testing should have his or her blood pressure checked again at regular intervals. A diastolic blood pressure that remains >90 mmHg is usually considered high blood pressure. This is often easily treated. To treat high blood pressure, it is important to know which medication a patient is taking and the possible side effects.

Heart attack is the nation's number-one killer, accounting for ~550,000 deaths each year. Heart attack usually occurs as a result of atherosclerosis, although it can be a result of a sudden abnormal heart rhythm or of a spasm of the arteries supplying the heart. *Three of every four heart attacks occur after the age of 65.* If a patient has had a heart attack, it is important to ask about the symptoms that preceded it, whether the patient has angina now, and how the angina is treated (rest, nitroglycerin, etc.)

Because blacks are almost 50 percent more likely than whites to have high blood pressure, they suffer an increased risk of heart attack and stroke. Younger women are much less likely than men to have heart attacks. After menopause, however, the risk of heart attack for women begins to increase, reaching that of men ~10 years after menopause.

Family members of patients at high risk should be encouraged to seek training in basic cardiac life support (BCLS). Some Heart Association affiliates have established specific training programs for family members of patients at high risk. Therapists and patients should contact their local American Heart Association affiliate for further details.

SYSTEM ENTRY

Therapists must be prepared to respond appropriately and immediately to a medical emergency that occurs while a patient is in their care, in order to prevent a sudden accident or illness from becoming a catastrophe. Whether in a hospital, a long-term care facility, or a patient's home, the therapist must know how to activate the emergency medical services (EMS) system. Hospitals and long-term care facilities usually have written procedures and protocols to follow in cases of medical emergencies. The therapist must be thoroughly familiar with the procedures. If there are no written guidelines, the therapist in a private home must be sure to keep the following information readily available (the therapist should keep this information at hand at all times for each patient.):

1. *Emergency numbers*
   Emergency medical (ambulance)
   Fire
   Police
   Physician (Office and home numbers)
2. Location of the nearest hospital emergency room that provides *24-hour* emergency cardiac care.
3. *Early warning signs* of a medical emergency. For patients in your care, you must be able to recognize these signs and provide the immediate care needed to sustain life until a rescue team or unit arrives. When you make the call to activate the EMS system, tell them:
   Where the emergency is, with cross streets if possible
   The phone number you are calling from
   What has happened
   How many people need help
   Condition of the patient(s)

Much of this information can be obtained from the patient or patient's family. You hang up *last* (let the person you called hang up first).

CARDIAC EMERGENCIES

Recognition

Early recognition of and intervention in cases of cardiac emergencies is the key to the survival of the patient. More than 50 percent of all heart attack victims die outside the hospital, most within 2 hours of the initial symptoms. The most significant symptom of a heart attack in persons <65 years of age is chest pain. The chest pain (angina pectoris) is caused by a poor supply of oxygen to the heart muscle. The pain or discomfort may be described as uncomfortable pressure, squeezing, fullness or tightness, aching, crushing, or an oppressive or heavy weight. It is usually centrally located in the chest behind the breast bone, or may be more diffuse throughout the chest. The pain may radiate to one or both shoulders, arms, neck, jaw, or back. The pain or discomfort will usually last longer than 2 minutes, and it may come and go. Other signs may be any or all of the following: sweating, nausea, shortness of breath, and/or a general feeling of weakness. The therapist should keep in mind that for the elderly the pain may not be severe and the patient may not look terribly ill. Physical or emotional stress are not necessarily precipitating factors of heart attack.

The patient's first tendency is to deny the possibility of heart attack, which further inhibits early intervention. It is incumbent on the therapist to recognize any warning signs and take the appropriate action. It is crucial to remember that among the elderly, symptoms are usually unique to each patient; however, a patient who experienced only slight dizziness and shortness of breath with a first heart attack must be alerted to the fact that another heart attack may or may not manifest the same symptoms. It is important to take all symptoms seriously, and the patient should be encouraged to report all symptoms.

Emergency Care

Once the therapist recognizes the signs and symptoms of a possible cardiac emergency, the patient should be made to stop all activity and rest calmly and quietly. The patient should be allowed to assume a position either lying down or sitting up that allows the most comfort and ease of breathing. If the patient's typical chest pain or other discomfort lasts for ≥2 minutes, the therapist should activate the EMS system. If an ambulance is not available, the patient should be taken immediately to the nearest hospital emergency room that provides 24-hour emergency cardiac care. If the patient has a known history of heart disease and has instructions from a physician to take nitroglycerin tablets (under the tongue), this procedure should be repeated at 3- to 5-minute intervals to a total dose of three tablets. If discomfort is not relieved and symptoms persist for 10 minutes despite rest and three nitroglycerin tablets, the EMS system should be activated. If an ambulance is not available, the patient should be taken immediately to the nearest hospital emergency room that provides 24-hour emergency cardiac care. The therapist must be sure to monitor the patient continuously and must be prepared to provide BCLS as necessary.

Cardiac Arrest

Cardiac arrest (the abrupt, unexpected cessation of breathing and circulation) may occur as the initial and only manifestation of coronary artery disease or may occur in individuals with known coronary disease. There are numerous noncardiac causes for cardiac arrest, including drowning, hypothermia, allergic reactions, electrocution, suffocation, major trauma, and stroke. In every case of cardiac arrest, time is critical. There is usually enough oxygen in the bloodstream and lungs to support life for up to 4 minutes when brain tissue begins to die. When breathing stops first, the heart will continue to pump for several minutes. When the heart stops, oxygen in the lungs and bloodstream can no longer be circulated to the vital organs. Victims whose heart and breathing have been interrupted for <4 minutes have an excellent chance for full recovery. After 6 minutes, however, significant brain damage occurs. The sooner circulation to the brain is restored, the greater the chance for full recovery.

Resuscitation

Cardiopulmonary resuscitation (CPR) is the method used to restore breathing and circulation. CPR combines artificial respiration or rescue breathing and manual compression of the heart. CPR at best provides 25 to 30 percent of normal circulation, which serves to place the patient in a holding pattern until normal breathing and circulation can be restored. The survival of the patient in cardiac arrest as well as survival without brain deficit is dependent on some-one who knows how to perform CPR being on the scene within 1 to 2 minutes. To learn CPR, one must attend a formal class that allows the participant sufficient supervised training in the psychomotor skill of CPR. CPR is learned in terms of:

1.   Sequence (what to do when);
2.   Timing (the minimum and maximum time allowed for each step); and
3.   Critical performance (actions that are critical to perform and key to each of the steps performed).

As in all fields of medicine, constant improvements are made in CPR techniques as more and more data become available and as research is done. The new standards for BCLS were published in *The Journal of the American Medical Association* in June 9, 1986. It is important that professionals in all health care fields continue to update their knowledge as these changes are approved.

The three primary areas of concern in performing CPR are

Airway—establishing a patent airway
Breathing—establishing rescue breathing
Circulation—restoring some level of circulation through manual compression of the heart.

The basic approach to the patient and steps in performing CPR can be reviewed as a part of summoning the ambulance after patient information has been given. Information about correct performance of CPR should be carried by the therapist at all times.

Resuscitation Adaptations for the Elderly

In performing CPR for the elderly patient, several factors and possible concerns should be considered.

Checking for Responsiveness

In checking for responsiveness, the therapist should use both sound and tactile (touch) stimulation because the patient may have difficulty in hearing/seeing.

Opening the Airway

Several methods are acceptable for opening the airway. The head-tilt chin-lift method is clearly the method of choice for the elderly patient. The therapist opens the airway by placing the fingers of one hand on the bony portion of the patient's lower jaw near the chin and lifting so as to bring the chin forward. This supports the jaw and helps tilt the head back. Caution must be taken to avoid applying any pressure to the soft tissue area under the chin, thereby occluding the airway. The hand closest to the head of the patient presses on the patient's forehead to tilt the head back. In this method, the chin is lifted so that the teeth are nearly brought together. Care should be taken to avoid complete closing of the mouth. This method supports the patient's lower jaw, bringing the teeth almost to occlusion, and maintains the position of loose dentures. Dentures should not be removed unless they cannot be managed in place.

The head-tilt neck-lift method is no longer an acceptable method for opening the airway and should not be used. It does not allow management of dentures, and excess force in performing this maneuver may cause cervical spine injury.

Rigidity of the neck may also complicate opening the airway of the elderly patient, making it impossible for the therapist to tilt the patient's head without incurring risk of cervical spine injury in the patient. (This is a special problem with all patients with a forward or flexed posture). If resistance in tilting the head back is encountered, the therapist should not tilt the head but should use the jaw thrust method either without tilting the head or, if possible without too much force, with a moderate head tilt. If the patient has a suspected neck or back injury, the therapist should use the jaw thrust maneuver without the head tilt to open the patient's airway.

Determining Absence of Breathing

To determine if the patient is breathing, the therapist places an ear next to the patient's mouth and nose and faces the patient's chest, watching the chest to see if it is rising and falling, listening for the return flow of the air during exhalation, and feeling for the flow of air. If the patient's chest does not rise and fall and there is no sound of exhaled air or feel of flow of exhaled air, the patient is breathless. Determination of whether the patient is breathing cannot be made by chest movement alone. The therapist must assess whether there is air movement in and out of the chest. The rigidity of the chest of the elderly patient often makes determination of breathlessness more difficult.

Rescue Breathing

If the patient is not breathing, the rescuer should call someone to help and should give the patient 2 slow full ventilations (1–1.5 second/inspiration). Mouth-to-mouth breathing provides the necessary oxygen to sustain life. Rescue breathing requires that the therapist, as the rescuer, inflate the patient's lungs adequately with each breath, assessing this by watching the chest. The patient's chest is sufficiently inflated when it rises. When rescue breathing is performed, the open airway must be maintained and an airtight seal must be created. The thumb and index finger of the hand maintaining the head tilt may be used to gently seal the nostrils of the patient by pinching them. As the rescuer, one takes a breath and seals the patient's lips with one's lips around the outside of the patient's mouth. Air is blown into the patient's mouth until the chest rises.

1. If the patient has no teeth and no dentures or has serious facial injuries, it may be necessary to use mouth-to-nose breathing. One hand is used to tilt the patient's head back and the other hand is used to lift the patient's lower jaw and close the mouth. As the rescuer, one takes a deep breath and seals the patient's nostrils with one's own lips, blows until the patient's chest rises, removes one's mouth, and opens the patient's mouth to allow exhalation.

2. *Some patients who require rescue breathing may have undergone a laryngectomy* (surgical removal of the larynx) and have a permanent stoma (an opening in the front base of the neck that connects the trachea with the skin). One makes a seal with the mouth over the stoma and blows until the chest rises, then removes one's mouth from the stoma, allowing the patient to exhale.

3. *A patient may have a temporary tracheostomy* (tube in the trachea). One ventilates these patients by sealing the patient's mouth and nose and blowing in the tube until the chest rises. The rescuer's mouth is removed from the tube and the patient is allowed to exhale. Some patients may have a cuff attached to the tube that can be inflated and will serve to seal the nose and mouth. If a cuff is present it is simply inflated and air is blown through the tube until the chest rises.

4. Rescue breathing can cause *gastric distention*. This usually occurs when the stomach limits chest ventilation volumes to the point at which the chest rises. Marked distention may promote regurgitation and reduce lung volume by elevating the diaphragm. If the patient's stomach becomes distended, the rescuer must recheck and reposition the airway and carefully observe the chest rise and fall to avoid excess ventilation pressure. Rescue breathing should be continued without any attempt made to expel the patient's stomach contents. *If regurgitation occurs, the patient should be turned on one side and the entire mouth should be wiped out,* the body returned to supine position and CPR continued. If severe gastric distention results in inadequate ventilation that is not corrected by repositioning the airway and reducing ventilation pressure, the patient is turned on one side and pressure is gently applied over the epigastrium (middle upper portion of the abdomen) to expel the air. Continuous pressure should never be maintained on the abdomen during CPR to prevent gastric distention. There is a danger of trapping the liver and possibly rupturing it. This could also cause the patient to regurgitate and aspirate the stomach contents.

Immediately after giving two full ventilations, determine if the patient is pulseless. This is done by palpating the carotid artery. (If the patient has moderate to severe coronary artery occlusion on one side that makes it difficult to take a pulse, one must be sure to adapt monitoring of the pulse as is needed.) The head tilt is maintained with one hand on the forehead; the other hand locates the carotid pulse on the side closest to the rescuer. The patient's larynx (voice box) is located with two fingers, sliding these fingers into the groove on the side between the trachea and the muscle at the side of the neck. The rescuer should avoid putting pressure on both carotid arteries at the same time as this could obstruct the blood flow to the brain. If the *pulse is present* and there is *no breathing,* rescue breathing is continued 12 times per minute or once every 5 seconds and EMS is activated. If the patient is breathing and has a pulse, the rescuer maintains the airway, continues to monitor vital signs, and activates EMS. A patient who has no pulse and no breathing is given chest compressions at a rate of 80 to 100 per minute (15 per 9–11 seconds), with two breaths given after every 15 chest compressions. The patient's pulse is checked after the first minute and every few minutes thereafter.

It is important to get professional help as soon as possible. If the rescuer is alone and the patient is in cardiac arrest and no one is nearby, the rescuer must begin CPR and continue for a period of 1 minute, then activate the EMS system and continue CPR.

In performing external chest compressions, proper hand position is especially important in the elderly patient. (Information of proper hand position should be part of the CPR information carried with the therapist). The fragility of the surrounding ribs will lead to fractures and soft tissue injury, if proper hand position is not maintained. Laceration of the liver by the xiphoid process may also result.

In all patients, the possibility of rib fractures, fracturing of the sternum, etc., exists. The elderly patient is at greater risk for these occurrences. If CPR must be performed for the elderly patient, close attention must be paid to correct hand position and body position, and compressions must be smooth and even. If rib fractures occur, the therapist must recheck hand position and continue CPR.

Only in the following instances may one stop CPR once one has initiated it:

The patient regains normal pulse and breathing
Another trained individual takes over
Physician or physician-directed team or person takes over
A person properly trained in EMS takes over
One is too exhausted to continue

Decision to Resuscitate

The decision of whether or not BCLS should be initiated for the elderly patient in cardiac arrest is a decision that should be made consciously in consultation with the patient, family members and the physician if the possibility of cardiac arrest exists. This should be discussed in advance. When the therapist is in doubt, CPR should be initiated.

RESPIRATORY EMERGENCIES

Anything that interferes with the normal breathing process or creates an insufficiency of oxygen in the blood is considered a respiratory emergency. The following are signs of a respiratory emergency:

1. No chest movement or uneven chest movement
2. No air felt or heard at the mouth and nose or exchange of air that is below normal
3. Noisy, shallow, or labored breathing
4. Gray or blue skin color

Airway Obstruction

The most common respiratory emergency is airway obstruction. Foreign body airway obstruction usually occurs during eating and a piece of meat is most often the cause. The elderly patient is quite susceptible to airway obstruction because dentures and poorly chewed food are common factors in foreign body obstruction. After suffering a stroke, patients often have difficulty swallowing. Poorly fitting dentures should be replaced, and teeth should be cared for to facilitate ease of chewing.

An unconscious patient can develop an airway obstruction when the tongue falls backward and blocks the airway. Regurgitation during cardiac arrest and blood clots resulting from facial injuries can also obstruct the airway in the unconscious patient.

Foreign bodies can cause either full or partial airway obstruction. Early recognition of foreign body obstruction is important. In cases of partial obstruction, the patient may have good air exchange or poor air exchange: If the patient is breathing adequately and can speak, there is good air exchange. If the patient cannot cough adequately and cannot speak and is turning blue, the air exchange is not sufficient to sustain life. A partial obstruction with poor air exchange should be managed in the same way as a full obstruction. The patient with a partial obstruction with good air exchange should be encouraged to cough. The normal coughing reflex that occurs in these cases is the best way to relieve an obstruction. This person must not be slapped on the back because a slap could cause a partial obstruction with poor air exchange. Therapists should refer to techniques taught in their CPR certification course.

Respiratory Failure

Respiratory failure is either the cessation of normal breathing or the reduction of breathing to the point at which oxygen intake is insufficient to sustain life. Respiratory arrest is cessation of breathing. Central respiratory arrest occurs when any condition exists that depresses or destroys the respiratory center in the brain. Some common causes of inadequate blood supply to the brain that can cause respiratory arrest are stroke, cardiac arrest, heart attack, and drug overdose. Head trauma, disease, or injuries that interfere with the normal contraction of the muscles of the respiratory system also cause respiratory emergencies. The emergency care for respiratory emergencies for the elderly patient is as follows:

1.   The respiratory emergency is recognized.
2.   The patient is placed in the position that will best facilitate breathing (sitting up or lying down with shoulders and chest raised). If unconscious, the patient is placed on the side, knees flexed, head resting on arm raised over the head on the side closest to the ground (if flexibility allows) or supported by an article as thick as the patient's upper arm. The patient's airway is open.
3.   The EMS system is activated.
4.   The patient is monitored to assure that respiratory arrest does not occur before help arrives.
5.   Basic life support/cardiopulmonary resuscitation is performed as symptoms require.

MEDICAL EMERGENCIES

The term medical emergencies is used to refer to illness or sickness resulting from a deficiency in structure or function of an organ or to disease caused by an infectious organism or the effect of a harmful substance. A medical emergency can be chronic, episodic, or acute, and can be life-threatening. In some cases, a medical emergency may occur in conjunction with an injury. Prompt recognition of a medical emergency, patient assistance, and appropriate emergency care can save a life. One should assume that a medical emergency exists if the patient's general state of health appears to be unusual, the patient's vital signs are atypical, or if the patient complains of feeling not "normal." (All patient complaints should be considered valid). The therapist must be aware of any chronic or episodic medical problems that the patient being treated may have.

Stroke

Stroke, also known as cerebrovascular accident (CVA), occurs when blood supply to the brain is interrupted either by a clot or by disruption of a blood vessel supplying the brain.

Elderly patients with high blood pressure, a cardiac history, and/or those who smoke heavily are high-risk candidates for a stroke.

Signs and symptoms of a stroke can include sudden weakness or paralysis of one or both sides of the body, inability to speak or communicate, loss of vision or double vision, unequal pupils, and loss of bladder control.

First aid treatment for the stroke victim should include the following:

1. Make sure the person is breathing adequately.
    a. Position a patient who is not having problems with the airway (no secretions or "snoring"), head and shoulders slightly elevated;
    b. If the breathing is *very shallow and slow,* mouth-to-mouth resuscitation may be indicated.
    c. If the breathing is accompanied by a "snoring" type of sound, tilt the patient's head back in order to displace the tongue from the upper airway. If breathing is hampered by vomitus or other secretions, turn the patient to the side and clear the mouth; continue mouth-to-mouth resuscitation.
2. Prevent loss of the patient's body heat but do not overheat;
3. *Do not* give the patient anything to eat or drink;
4. Reassure the patient. Remember, just because the person may not be able to talk, he or she may not be unaware of what is going on or what is being said.
5. Activate the EMS system.

Diabetic Emergencies

Body cells need glucose (sugar) for normal functioning and energy. To utilize the glucose in the human body, a substance called insulin is required. Diabetes seriously interferes with the ability of the body to utilize sugar owing to deficiencies in insulin production.

When glucose increases to abnormal levels in the blood supply, hyperglycemia develops. Signs and symptoms of hyperglycemia include frequent urination, increased thirst, and sugar in the urine. Hyperglycemia is caused by diabetics failing to take their prescribed amounts of insulin, unusual amounts of stress, or infection that is left untreated. This condition can gradually lead to diabetic coma. Diabetic coma is a life-threatening condition, signs and symptoms of which may include the following:

1. Signs and symptoms of hyperglycemia
2. Gradual onset
3. Rapid, deep breathing with a sweet or acetone breath odor
4. Rapid, weak pulse
5. Red, dry skin
6. Abdominal pain
7. Fever

On the other hand, insulin shock, or hypoglycemia, results when a diabetic has too much insulin, usually caused by insufficient food, excessive stress or exercise, exposure to cold, or taking more than the prescribed dose of insulin.

The signs and symptoms of insulin shock can include the following:

1. Sudden onset
2. Extreme weakness
3. Pale, moist skin
4. Shallow breathing
5. Rapid pulse
6. Altered mental state (appearing confused, disoriented)

Any person who is a diabetic and who either shows signs of or complains of symptoms resembling either diabetic coma or insulin shock should be cared for in the following manner:

If the victim is unconscious:

1. Lay the victim flat on the side and keep the airway open.
2. Do not try to give the victim anything by mouth.

If the victim is conscious:

1. Place the victim in a comfortable position.
2. Ask whether the victim has taken insulin or eaten.
3. Give candy or any sweetened fruit juice; if coughing reflex is present, this will usually quickly reverse hypoglycemic states.

It may be difficult to recognize the differences between diabetic coma and insulin shock; thus administration of sugar is recommended for any diabetic who appears ill or acts abnormally. Although giving sugar to a person in diabetic coma adds little risk of seriously worsening the person's condition, it may save the life or prevent brain damage of the person in insulin shock.

In all cases of either diabetic coma or insulin shock, treat for shock and get medical assistance immediately.

Seizure

Seizures represent sudden changes in muscle activity or behavior owing to an "electrical storm" in the brain. A person having a seizure has no control over his or her actions.

Causes of seizures can include fever (especially in small children), head injury, alcohol, and a host of other physical problems. When the problem cannot be pinpointed, the person is classified as having epilepsy.

The type of seizure can range from brief periods of staring, usually occurring in children (petit mal seizures) to alternating contraction and relaxation of all extremities (grand mal seizure). Components of a seizure include the following:

1. Aura, a sensation that precedes and sometimes warns the victim that a seizure is imminent
2. Loss of consciousness
3. Continuous muscle contraction
4. Rhythmic contraction and relaxation of muscles
5. A drowsy or "sleep-like" state
6. Confused, disoriented, thrashing, combative state

Emergency care for a seizure should include the following:

1. *Stay calm.*
2. Make sure the airway is controlled.
3. Stay with the victim until the seizure passes.
4. Make sure the head and body are protected from injury during the seizure by putting a pillow or blanket under the head and moving furniture away from the victim.
5. Loosen tight clothing.
6. Do not try to hold the victim down; this may lead to fractured bones.
7. Ask the "curious" to leave the scene of the seizure.
8. Allow the victim to rest after the seizure and offer reassurance. If there is a known history of seizures, when the person becomes lucid ask whether professional medical assistance is desired.
9. If the seizure lasts more than 3 to 5 minutes or the victim goes into a second seizure, have an ambulance called immediately.

Chronic Obstructive Pulmonary Disease

Chronic obstructive pulmonary disease (COPD) includes chronic bronchitis, emphysema, and other respiratory emergencies that are similar to emphysema. Medical emergencies related to COPD generally affect the older patient who may have a current or past history of heavy smoking, a persistent cough, tightness in the chest, periods of dizziness in some cases, cyanosis, and/or edema of the lower extremities. They wish to sit upright, have a barrel-chest appearance and wheeze, and breathe in puffs holding their lips tight.
Emergency care for COPD is as follows:

1. Assure an open airway and monitor vital signs.
2. Allow patient to assume position of greatest comfort.
3. Loosen any restrictive clothing.
4. Maintain normal body temperature.
5. Reduce stress as much as possible (help person feel safe and in control of the situation).

6. If oxygen is available, administer at 24 percent by Venturi mask (usually 100 percent oxygen at 2 to 5 L/min delivers 24 percent, or follow patient's instructions).

7. Activate EMS system immediately.

Acute Abdominal Distress

Underlying cause of acute abdominal distress for the elderly patient can be intestinal obstruction, strangulated hernia, inflammation of the pancreas, inflammation of the abdominal cavity membranes (peritonitis), diverticulitis, or ulcers. It may be no more than indigestion. Occasionally heart attacks begin as abdominal pain rather than chest pain. The patient with an acute abdomen has many different signs and symptoms including:

1. Localized or diffuse pain and tenderness of the abdomen (with or without guarding)
2. Nausea, vomiting, diarrhea, or constipation
3. Rapid pulse and low blood pressure
4. Rapid shallow breathing, response to pain
5. Fever
6. Soft or rigid, or distended abdomen; there may be a protrusion
7. Possible bleeding from the rectum or vagina, or blood in the urine

Emergency care for the patient with an acute abdomen is as follows:

1. Maintain open airway and monitor vital signs.
2. Be on the alert for vomiting.
3. Position the patient on the side or back with knees flexed.
4. Do not give the patient anything by mouth.
5. Maintain body temperature.
6. Activate the EMS system immediately.

Communicable Diseases

A patient may have a communicable disease if fever, profuse sweating, nausea, vomiting, rapid pulse, shallow breathing, nontraumatic stiffness of neck or chest, abdominal pain, rash, headaches, coughing, and sneezing are present.

Emergency care for a patient with a communicable disease is as follows:

1. Maintain the airway and monitor vital signs.
2. Maintain body temperature.
3. Allow the patient to assume the position of most comfort.
4. Activate the EMS system.
5. Protect yourself from contamination during care of the patient. Consult

the emergency department physician or the patient's physician regarding directions for personal care, disposal, cleaning, and sterilization of equipment and supplies.

Poisoning, Drug, and Alcohol-Related Emergencies

A poison is any liquid, solid, or gas that impairs health or causes death when it is introduced into the body through ingestion (through the stomach), inhalation (through the lungs), absorption (through the skin) or injection.

Ingested Poisons

In general, the principles of emergency care of a patient suffering from an ingested poison are to maintain the patient's airway and to call the local area Poison Control Center for further advice. For example, in New York City, the Poison Control Center can be reached by dialing P-O-I-S-O-N-S. The following information will be needed by the Poison Control Center or physician in order to issue specific instructions:

1. Age of victim
2. Name of poison
3. Amount of poison swallowed and when (if known)
4. The first aid being given and whether the victim has vomited
5. The present location of the victim and how long it will take to get to the victim a hospital
6. The label and/or container of poison (these should be saved)
7. Vomitus, if any; bring it to the hospital with you. In case the Poison Control Center cannot be reached, it is safe to dilute the poison by giving the patient either water or milk if the victim is conscious and not convulsing. Do not induce vomiting in an unconscious patient or if the patient has ingested a corrosive chemical.

Do not neutralize the poison with vinegar or lemon juice.
Do not give oils.
As a rule, vomiting should never be induced in an unconscious person or in a person who has ingested strong acid, strong alkali, or petroleum products. In a situation in which vomiting should be induced, administration of syrup of ipecac is the method of choice. Follow the directions on the label.

Inhaled Poisons

The most common inhaled gas that causes poisoning is carbon monoxide (CO), a tasteless, odorless, colorless gas. Carbon monoxide is present in the exhaust fumes of cars, lanterns, and sewer gas, and is a common product of fires confined to a small space. The initial symptoms include headache, weakness, dizziness, shortness of breath, and a cherry red appearance of the skin.

Other common inhaled poisons include carbon dioxide, ammonia, and chlorine gas.

The first step to take is to get the patient into a normal breathing environment. If the rescuer cannot do this alone, the local police or fire department should be called.

When brought to safety, the victim should be checked for signs of ventilation. If ventilation is absent, rescue breathing should be started immediately. A victim who is breathing adequately should be allowed to rest. An ambulance should be called.

Absorbed Poisons (Contact Poisons)

Many substances can be absorbed directly through the skin in large enough quantities to be poisonous. The most common among these are harsh chemicals, corrosives, and toxins produced by plants.

Harsh chemicals, corrosives, and pesticides can produce chemical skin burns and require immediate treatment. The burned area should be flushed continously with water until help arrives.

Some plants, such as poison ivy, poison sumac, and poison oak, can cause marked allergic reactions on contact with the skin. This reaction is characterized by redness, itching, rash, swelling, and blisters, and can be accompanied by headaches and fever.

Emergency care of patients suffering from absorbed poisons is as follows:

1. Wearing gloves, remove the victim's contaminated clothing and flush the area with a large amount of tepid water for at least 20 minutes.
2. If the poison is either corrosive or a pesticide, send for an ambulance.
3. If the patient is unconscious, keep the airway open, provide BCLS as necessary and treat for shock.
4. In cases of pesticides or unusual poisons, save the label of the container or a sample of the vomitus.
5. Wash any area of your skin that comes in contact with the poison.
6. If the contact poison is a plant, flush the skin with large amounts of water and scrub with soap and water for at least 5 minutes. After washing, apply rubbing alcohol and calamine or other soothing lotion.
7. Get medical help if there is a severe reaction to contact with the plant.

Alcohol Abuse

Alcohol is a depressant, initially creating a feeling of relaxation or exhilaration and later causing disruption in motor activity, motor skills, and coordination. Respirations may decrease; the patient may lose consciousness, resulting in coma or death.

The emergency care for alcohol abuse is as follows:

1. If the patient is sleeping, and his coloring, breathing, and pulse are normal, no emergency care is necessary.
2. If signs of shock are present, immediate care is necessary.
3. Maintain an open airway.
4. Apply CPR as necessary.
5. Treat for shock.
6. Activate the EMS system.

Drug Abuse/Drug Overdose/Drug–Drug Interaction

A drug is a substance that affects body functions or the mind when taken into the body or applied to the body surface. Drug abuse is the persistent use of a drug without regard to accepted medical practice. This can manifest itself as a patient who takes certain over-the-counter medications in combination with medically prescribed medication or who borrows someone else's medication. A drug overdose can occur when a patient accidently mistakes one medication bottle for another or, owing to short-term memory problems, constantly takes a larger dose than is prescribed. Last, among the elderly, drug–drug interaction may occur when a patient takes an old medication (saved from a previous problem) and forgets to tell the physician, who prescribes a drug, and the old medication may alter the body's reaction to the new medication.

In cases of drug abuse, drug overdose, or drug–drug reaction, emergency care should be provided as follows:

If the patient is conscious

1. Reassure and protect the patient.
2. Protect yourself and others in the area.
3. Get medical assistance.
4. "Talk the patient down," (create a sense of safety and control for the patient) if the drug is a hallucinogen.

If the patient is unconscious:

1. Maintain an open airway.
2. Give basic life support/cardiopulmonary resuscitation as necessary.
3. Treat for shock.
4. Obtain medical help immediately.
5. Try to arouse the patient if the drug is a narcotic, depressant, or tranquilizer.

Information that will be helpful to a physican or drug abuse treatment center include:

1. Type of drug(s) (prescription and nonprescription)
2. Age and size of patient
3. General condition of the patient

One must bear in mind that *more* than one drug may have been taken and apply the general principles for emergency treatment. It is not unusual for an elderly patient to be on five different medications at one time.

The elderly patient may have difficulty remembering whether or not they have taken the medication(s). Work with the physician to establish a check system for the patient to avoid taking medication(s) twice or at the wrong times.

Anaphylactic Shock

When a person comes in contact with something to which he or she is extremely allergic, anaphylactic shock may ensue. This is the most severe form of an allergic reaction. The blood vessels and other tissues are affected directly by the allergic reaction. Commonly, the victim develops hives and red, hot, itchy skin. Within a few minutes, blood pressure falls, and severe shortness of breath develops owing to swelling of respiratory passages and tongue. If the victim is left untreated, swelling in the air passage may block the airway. This form of shock can become life-threatening very quickly. It is important to obtain medical assistance immediately.

Substances that most commonly cause allergic reactions fall into the following groups:

1. Injections—eg, penicillin
2. Insect stings—bee, wasp, hornet, or yellow jacket
3. Ingestion—fish, shellfish, berries, or certain drugs
4. Inhalation—pollens, ragweed, dust, and dander

It is important to remember that any food, medication, or material can cause an allergic reaction. Patients with a history of allergies or anaphylactic shock should be advised to use a system for recording their allergies/and possible self-administered treatment (ie, epinephrine injection) that will be accessible to emergency personnel (ie, Medic Alert bracelet or Vial of Life label on refrigerator).

ENVIRONMENTAL EMERGENCIES

Our environment is a delicate balance of many factors that allow human life to exist as we know it. Occasionally, humans are exposed to extremes of these factors, the result of which causes a disruption of the organism's internal workings. We can anticipate some of the possible effects of these extremes and learn how to react to them. The elderly patient is very susceptible to environmental changes. Vulnerability to heat extremes is also enhanced by diuretic therapy, phenothiazines, inability to obtain fluid appropriately (eg, bedbound), a move from hot or cold environment, and mind-altering substances.

Exposure to Heat

The exposure of the body to extremes of heat may be manifested in ways other than burns. Heat-related emergencies are divided into three categories: heat cramps, heat exhaustion, and heat stroke.

Heat Cramps

Heat cramps may occur in the healthiest of individuals. They usually affect people who are working in a hot environment and perspiring profusely. Usually characterized by severe muscle cramps in the legs and/or abdomen, heat cramps are often accompanied by exhaustion to the point of collapse with some dizziness and possible fainting.

More than 70 percent of the human body is water in which various substances are dissolved. One of these substances, salt, is in critical balance with water, and normal muscular action depends on this balance. Salt, not just water, must be taken in, or an imbalance will occur in the muscle tissues, causing the involuntary spasms of heat cramps. Therefore, the most effective treatment for the relief of heat cramps is sips of salt water (one teaspoon of salt to one quart of water). In conjunction with administration of salt water, the patient should be removed to a cool place, and the cramped muscle should be massaged. Although apparently not in serious condition, the victim of heat cramps should be given immediate follow-up medical attention.

Heat Exhaustion

The effects of physical exertion in a hot environment can be more generalized and severe. In an attempt to maintain normal temperature, the body reacts to heat by transporting blood from its interior core to the skin. There the heat escapes to cooler surroundings by radiation and conduction. This movement of blood to the skin, in addition to the pooling of blood in the lower extremities if the person is standing for long periods, may lead to an inadequate return of blood to the heart and brain, resulting in physical collapse. Such a condition is called heat exhaustion (prostration), and essentially is another form of shock.

Signs and symptoms of heat exhaustion include a weak pulse; rapid, shallow breathing; general weakness; pale, clammy skin; profuse perspiration; dizziness; and, in some cases, unconsciousness.

Heat exhaustion is treated in the same manner as shock, with the exception of covering the victim. In addition, as much heat is removed as possible by moving the victim to a cooler environment, removing as much clothing as possible, and fanning the victim. Be careful to avoid overcooling the victim; remember, we want to restore normal body temperature (98.6°F). The EMS system must always be activated in these cases, since associated changes in body chemistry will need to be evaluated and corrected immediately.

Heat Stroke

If the conditions described for heat exhaustion persist, either in the environment or in the body, the body's mechanism for dissipating excess heat may be overwhelmed. If the body's ability to perspire shuts down and heat continues to build up in the body to a point at which cells, particularly in the brain, are permanently damaged, this condition is defined as *heat stroke*. Because of its lethal potential, it is considered a *true emergency* and requires immediate attention at a medical facility. A rescuer who calls for an ambulance must be sure to inform medical personnel that the victim has suffered heat stroke. (The elderly are more vulnerable, since it is common to have an alteration in the sweating response with advanced age.)

The symptoms of heat stroke are distinct from those of other heat emergencies. Heat stroke is characterized by deep breathing deteriorating to shallow respirations; rapid strong pulse deteriorating to rapid weak pulse; dry, hot skin; dilated pupils; convulsions; and loss of consciousness.

Treatment must be begun as soon as the patient's condition is recognized. Cool the patient in any manner possible and do it rapidly.

It can be accomplished in the following ways:

1.   Remove the patient from the source of heat. If the heat source is the sun, bring the victim into the shade.
2.   Remove as much of the victim's clothing as possible.
3.   Wrap the victim in towels dampened with cool water.
4.   If available, place ice packs under the victim's arms, on the wrists and ankles, and on either side of the neck.
5.   If transportation will be delayed, place the victim in a cold water bath. Never leave the victim alone in this bath.

Remember, heat stroke is a life-threatening emergency.

Exposure to Cold

The ill effects of cold on the human body are classified into two categories—local and generalized. Local cooling occurs in particular parts of the body, usually those inadequately protected from the environment; most commonly, these include the ears, nose, hands, and feet. As the result of exposure to extremely cold air or water, the blood supply to the area is limited due to constriction of the blood vessels; thus, the body is unable to maintain normal warmth. Frostbite, the common term used for this localized cooling, is progressive and, depending on the duration and degree of exposure, will cause progressive degrees of injury. For the purposes of this text, we will consider all frostbite as being the same.

The symptoms of frostbite begin as a reddening of the exposed skin. As exposure continues, the skin becomes gray or blotchy, with associated numbness. One should be aware, however, that tendons are resistant to freezing, and the patient will still be able to move the part. (Such movement should be discouraged.) When freezing eventually occurs, all sensation is lost, and the skin becomes dead white.

Treatment for frostbite should be done in the hospital.

First aid for frostbite should be as follows:

1. Remove any wet clothing.
2. Cover the affected area with dry clothing and keep the whole body warm and dry.
3. Give small amounts of warm fluids (*not coffee or other stimulants—* these cause further constriction of the blood vessels in the skin).
4. *Do not* massage or rub the affected area. Minimize all movement.

Generalized exposure to cold may cause core body temperature to decrease, leading to a state called *hypothermia.* As in heat stroke, the inability of the body to control its temperature constitutes a *true emergency.* The victim must be transported to a medical facility without delay.

Hypothermia may be recognized by shivering, feelings of numbness, drowsiness, slow breathing and pulse rates and, eventually, unconsciousness. The victim's mental state is the best measure of hypothermia, since even body temperatures between 95 to 96°F may be manifested by confused or withdrawn behavior.

Rewarming of the hypothermia victim should not be started until the patient is in the hospital. If done improperly, the rewarming process itself can produce life-threatening heart rhythms which, in this state, are not easily corrected. During the waiting or transporting time, the victim can be protected by removal of wet clothing and by being kept in a warm, dry environment. Because the body's mechanism for heat control is not functioning, simply wrapping the victim in blankets will be of little use. The victim should be placed in a warm environment, which the blankets will then help to maintain. Usually this will mean using external sources such as well-wrapped hot packs, hot water bottles, heating pads, or even a rescuer's body heat.

One must never assume that a victim of prolonged hypothermia is dead. Many cases of revival have been reported; therefore, every attempt at resuscitation should be made. The decision of death, by a physician, should only be made after the body temperature has been raised to a normal level consistent with life.

SURGICAL EMERGENCIES

Shock

The basic feature of shock, regardless of its origin, is an insufficient supply (perfusion) of oxygenated blood through the tissues of the body. In a shock state, the tissues are deprived of their normal supply of oxygen and nutrients, and the ability to eliminate waste materials is diminished.

Shock is a true medical emergency. If the precipitating causes are not treated, death soon ensues. Shock may be seen in cases of severe injury and serious illness. In some cases, prolonged and untreated less serious conditions may manifest the characteristics of shock.

The management of shock takes precedence over other emergencies exclusive of respiratory and/or cardiac arrest and severe or uncontrolled bleeding. The shock syndrome must be quickly corrected in order to prevent the deterioration of the patient.

General signs and symptoms of shock are as follows:

1. Restlessness and anxiety which may precede all other signs
2. A feeling of impending doom or disaster
3. A weak and rapid pulse, indicating decreased circulating blood volume and cardiac output
4. Pale, cold, and wet skin, often described as "clammy"; in the advanced stages of shock, the skin may appear blue, especially around the lips and nailbeds (this is known as cyanosis)
5. Shallow, irregular, labored, rapid or even gasping respirations. These fast, shallow respirations place a great demand on the respiratory muscles and require even more oxygen than is normally required.
6. Dull and lackluster eyes. The pupils may be dilated.
7. Extreme thirst
8. Nausea and possible vomiting
9. Dizziness and weakness
10. A gradual and steady fall in blood pressure, which may eventually be unobtainable. Some people have normally low blood pressure. Development of shock is suspected in an acutely injured adult with a systolic blood pressure of ≥ 100 mmHg.
11. Loss of consciousness

Care and Treatment of Shock

The treatment of shock is based primarily on prevention and early recognition. The "whole" victim must be considered; not just one or two problems.

Priority of treatment is as follows:

1. Secure and maintain a patent airway.

2. Control bleeding.

3. Elevate the lower extremities approximately 12 to 18 in. Do not tilt the entire body down, as this may interfere with respiration. This maneuver is not done in cases of head and chest injuries or profound injuries to the legs;

4. Immobilize any fractures.

5. Avoid rough and excessive handling of the victim in shock. *Shock can be aggravated by body movement.*

6. Prevent loss of body heat.

7. Keep the victim lying down in order to give the circulatory system a rest. For victims of a heart attack or breathing problem, a semisitting position will usually be more comfortable.

8. Do not give anything by mouth.

9. Record the victim's initial vital signs (blood pressure, pulse, respirations, temperature, etc.). Continue to monitor and record vital signs at 5-minute intervals until you are relieved by trained emergency medical personnel.

Soft Tissue Injuries

Recognition of the different types of soft tissue injuries and knowledge of their correct treatment is of utmost importance. Immediate action is required to control severe bleeding or the patient may perish in minutes. Minor soft tissue injuries with minimal bleeding still require care to prevent contamination of the wound and infection. Prompt and efficient treatment of specific types of wounds may prevent the necessity of hospitalization or significantly reduce the length of the patient's hospital stay.

There are two major categories of soft tissue injuries: closed and open wounds. For any wound, an immunization history must be taken, including the victim's most recent tetanus toxoid injection.

Whenever there is a break in the surface of the skin, an open wound is present. Open wounds range from a minor scrape, which may require little, if any, emergency treatment, to a complete loss of an extremity, which may require immediate emergency treatment to save life and limb.

There are two basic categories of bleeding: external and internal. These two categories can be further subdivided as to the origin of the bleeding: arterial (from the high-pressure vessels leading away from the heart); venous (from the low-pressure vessels leading to the heart and away from the body); and capillary (from small blood vessels that connect arteries to veins and in which oxygen and nutrient exchange between the blood and body occurs).

Emergency care for all types of internal bleeding consists of treatment for shock and rapid access to the EMS system.

External bleeding from an open wound can be treated immediately. The most serious type of external bleeding is arterial bleeding. It is possible for a patient to lose a large percentage of the total blood volume in a short period of time, causing death in a matter of minutes.

Three procedures are used to control bleeding: (1) direct pressure and elevation; (2) pressure points, and (3) only as a method of last resort, tourniquet.

Direct Pressure

The first method to use to control bleeding is application of pressure directly over the site of the wound. If a sterile dressing is immediately available, it should be placed over the wound and firm steady pressure should be applied to the wound. If there is no sign of spinal injury, extremity fractures, or embedded objects in the extremity, the extremity should be elevated. Raising the height of the extremity to a position higher than the level of the heart may reduce blood pressure in the veins and flow of blood from the vessel. Direct pressure is usually sufficient. Pressure should be maintained until appropriate medical personnel arrive.

Treatment of Open Wounds

The general rules to follow when treating open wounds are as follows:

1. Clear the wound surface—Cut away clothing from wound site and remove material from wound surface. Do not try to clean the wound or remove small particles within the wound itself.
2. Stop the bleeding—use direct pressure, elevation, and pressure points to control bleeding. A tourniquet should be used only as a last resort after all other methods have failed.
3. Cover the wound—apply a sterile dressing or clean handkerchief to prevent further contamination of the wound.

Treatment of Specific Types of Injuries

Impaled Objects

When a patient is stabbed by an object, ie, pick, knife, etc., and the object is not removed from the wound, it is said to be impaled. *Never remove an impaled object.* Movement of an impaled object may cause additional damage to underlying structures, such as arteries, veins, and nerves, thereby increasing bleeding or causing loss of nerve function. *Keep patient still until appropriate medical personnel arrives.*

Musculoskeletal Injuries

Injuries to bones, joints, and muscles result most often from falls in the elderly. These injuries are rarely emergencies requiring great speed in transportation, but great harm can be done if the victim is moved too hastily or handled too roughly.

Fractures, dislocations, and sprains exhibit many of the same signs and symptoms. It is impossible to determine at the scene the type of injury the victim may have sustained. Therefore, any suspected injury to bones and joints should be treated in a similar manner.

Suspect injury to bones and joints if:

1. The victim reports a history of a fall or other accident.
2. The victim cannot move the injured part.
3. The body part is deformed or discolored.
4. The body part is swollen or painful.
5. There seems to be abnormal movement in the area.
6. The victim has heard or felt the bone break.
7. An open wound is present at the site.

General principles of first aid for bone and joint injuries are:

1. *Do not move the victim* unless essential for safety. If the victim must be moved, pull or drag the victim to safety by the legs or the armpits along the long axis of the body.
2. Keep the airway open and give artificial respiration if needed.
3. Control severe bleeding by direct pressure and elevation.
4. Prevent movement of the injured part and adjacent joints.
5. Treat for shock.
6. Activate the EMS system.

Because most bone and joint injuries require ambulance transportation to a hospital, it is usually best not to attempt to splint or immobilize an injury but to wait for professional assistance. If medical help will be delayed and the victim must be transported, *always* apply splints before moving victim.

Do not attempt to move or splint any victim with an injury to the head, neck or back. It is always better to wait for help.

Burns

Burns are tissue injuries caused by heat, chemicals, electrical energy, and radiation.

All burn injuries require prompt emergency care. Severe burn injuries require medical care by a hospital equipped to care specifically for the burn patient. The immediate hazards of burns are: shock; swelling of tissues; swelling of tissues in the breathing passages; infection; loss of body fluids; disfigurement; loss of an eye, limb, or other part of the body; and death. Other hazards from fire include: inhalation of very hot poisonous gases; suffocation from too little oxygen in the air; and injuries from falls or collapsing parts of buildings.

The severity of a burn injury is determined by the *depth* of the burn; the *size* of the burn; and the *location* of the burn.

Burns are grouped into three degrees, but often it is difficult to tell immediately how deep a burn is, because swelling and blistering may appear 2 or 3 hours later.

Anyone who is burned may have a combination of various degrees of burns. Treatment should be given for the worst burn suspected.

Burns on the four critical areas of the body—*feet, face, hands and genital area*—are especially dangerous. Any second-degree burn or deeper burn on a critical area of the body, no matter how small, requires immediate medical attention. Burns of the face, nose, or mouth may indicate injury to the breathing passages. Injury of the breathing passages can result in swelling that can cause severe difficulty in breathing or block the breathing passages. Medical help must be obtained immediately, and the person should be watched to make sure that breathing continues. If breathing stops the victim must be given mouth-to-mouth resuscitation.

In addition to the depth, size, and location of the burn, the age and physical condition of the patient can contribute to the seriousness of burns.

Emergency Care for Burns

The major objectives of emergency care for burns are relief of pain, prevention of infection, and treatment for shock.

Small, Superficial Burns. Immerse the burn in cool water in order to reduce the pain. Gently pat the area dry with sterile gauze. It is not necessary to cover this type of burn unless it develops areas of blisters that need protection. If necessary, cover the burn with a dry, nonstick sterile dressing, and bandage the dressing in place.

Large, Superficial Burns. Cool the area with water immediately until the pain subsides. Dry it gently and cover it with a thick, dry, sterile dressing.

Deep Burns. Do not put water on an open burn to cool it. Water increases the chance of infection. Cover the burn with a thick, dry, sterile dressing and bandage. If burned clothing is sticking to the burn, place the dressing right over it. *Do not remove clothing that is sticking to the burn.* Do not wet the dressing. Have the person lie down, elevate the burn area, and seek medical help.

Heat Burns of the Eye. Gently flood water into any burn of the eye except a very deep burn. Examine the eye to see if a cinder or other object is loose on the surface of the eye. If there is an object loose on the surface, gently touch it out with the corner of a clean handkerchief or sterile dressing. Cover the eye with a thick, dry, sterile dressing, and bandage the dressing in place. If a cinder or other object is embedded in the eye, keep the eye from moving by bandaging both eyes. For deep burns of the eye, do not flood the eye with water. Bandage both eyes, place a cold pack over the bandaged eyes, elevate the head and shoulders, and give care for shock. *Get immediate medical care for any burn of the eye.*

Chemical Burns of the Skin.   Chemical burns occur when the skin comes in contact with corrosive materials. The burning process will continue as long as the solution remains in contact with the skin.

Immediately flush with water, using a shower or hose for at least 20 minutes; remove clothing that may have come in contact with the solution. Take the victim to the emergency room of a hospital, continuing irrigation en route. Give care for shock.

Note: wash all chemical burns and remove clothing from all chemical burns.

Chemical Burns of the Eye.   Acid and alkali burns can be caused by drain cleaner, strong laundry detergent, and other agents.

Flood the eye with water for 15 minutes. Have the person lie on one side and flood from the inner corner of the eye to the outer corner. Continue irrigation en route to the emergency room of the hospital. Cover the eye with a thick, dry, sterile dressing, and bandage it in place. If the eye is badly burned or something is embedded in the eye or eyelid, bandage both eyes to prevent eye movement. Get medical help immediately.

Shock in Burn Patients.   Shock, due to body fluid loss, is possible with any but the small, superficial burns. In shock, the functions of the body may become so depressed that a person may die.

Treat as previously described for shock.

Electrical Emergencies.   Electric shock may cause cardiac and respiratory arrest along with extensive burns.

Do not approach or touch the person suffering from electrical shock until you know it is safe to do so. Turn off the electrical current. If you cannot shut off the current, you may be able to roll the person away with one or two wooden poles, such as broom handles. Ropes or other materials that do not conduct electricity may be used. As soon as you rescue the person, check to see if there is a need to provide basic life support, check for other injuries, treat for shock, and get medical help.

SUMMARY

The basic tenets for dealing with a medical and/or surgical emergency of an elderly patient are the same as for any other patient. *Know your patient.* If an emergency occurs, remain calm. Remember to review CPR and stabilization techniques. Have emergency phone numbers immediately available and call for advice/help as soon as the patient is stable. When in doubt, call the primary care physician and/or access the EMS system. Appropriate help is always available.

SUGGESTED READINGS

Bedell SE, Delbanco TL, Cook EF, et al: Survival after cardiopulmonary resuscitation in the hospital. N Engl J Med 309(10):569, 1983

Gulati RS, Bhan GL, Horan MA: Cardiopulmonary resuscitation of old people. Lancet 2:267, 1983

Eisenberg MS, Hallstrom A, Bergner L: Long-term survival after out-of-hospital cardiac arrest. N Engl J Med 306:1340, 1982

Gordon M, Vadas P: Benefits of access to on-site acute and critical care for the residential section of a multi-level geriatric centre. A one-year review. J Am Geriatr Soc 32:453, 1984

Bedell SE, Delbanco TL. Choices about cardiopulmonary resuscitation in the hospital. N Engl J Med 310:1129, 1984

Wagner A: Cardiopulmonary resuscitation in the aged—a prospective study. N Engl J Med 310:1129, 1984

Herrin, TJ, Montgomery W: Instructors Manual for Basic Cardiac Life Support, American Heart Association, 1985

Breneman, JC, *Basics of Food Allergies,* Charles C. Thomas, Springfield, Ill, 1978

Grant H, Murray RH, Bergeron JD: Emergency Care. 3rd Ed. Brady, Bowie, Maryland, 1984

Hafen BQ: First Aid for Health Emergencies. 3rd Ed. West, St. Paul. Minn. 1985

American Heart Association Publications

Exercise Testing and Training of Apparently Healthy Individuals: A Handbook for Physicians. 1977

Exercise Testing and Training of Individuals with Heart Disease or at High Risk for its Development: A Handbook for Physicians. 1975

Exercise and Your Heart. 1984

An Older Person's Guide to Cardiovascular Health. 1983

9 | Environmental Assessment: Adaptations for Maximal Independence

Lena Karlqvist

The proportion of elderly people is increasing in most industrialized countries in the world. In particular, this demographic change affects the number of very old people. For example, in Sweden, the group of elderly >85 years of age is expected to double from 1970 to the year 2000 and the group ≥95 years of age is expected to triple. The situation is not very different in other western countries, and an increase of elderly is also expected in the developing countries of the world. According to a UN forecast, 350 million people in the developing world will be >60 years of age in the year 2000 as compared with ~230 million in the industrialized countries.

The increase of older people in society means a greater demand for care. However, this need is directly related to the health and functional status of each elderly person. Health status varies considerably among the elderly, and patterns of illness as well as functional losses are changing as the demographics of the elderly population change. Recent studies in Sweden reveal that there has been a successive vitalization of the elderly population over the past decades. The difference in activity level and functional abilities is noticeable even when comparisons are made between 70-year-old persons today and the same age group 5 years ago.[1]

On the average, women live longer than men. This fact becomes most noticeable among the group of elderly people who are >80 years of age and who require the most care. Hence, there is a preponderance of women in nursing homes, chronic care facilities, and in retirement homes. It appears likely that retirement homes and nursing homes should be governed by standards that reflect the needs and/or the desires of the majority of patients (women).

Our basic hypothesis is that the physical environment plays a crucial role in the well-being of the elderly person. The nursing home with its staff and assistive devices can provide an environment that stimulates the elderly and helps the patients to maintain their motivation and maximal independence in all activities. This chapter focuses on the crucial question: How should a geriatric unit in a hospital, nursing home, or the patients own home be organized in order to meet the needs of the elderly and still be able to provide a safe and reasonable working environment for the staff and/or family to assist the patient as needed?

A brief account of functional abilities of elderly persons is given so that basic environmental adaptations can be looked at from a perspective of preventive health care. For example, it is possible for a senior center to incorporate basic environmental adaptations to maximize independence and self-confidence and thereby create a truly therapeutic environment. The argument about environmental adaptations to maximize independence can also apply to the doctor's or physical therapist's office, the out-patient clinic, or the acute hospital room. A case study is presented in which an analysis of the environment is made of a typical patient room in a hospital or nursing home. The aspects of the environment that can cause a reduction in the functional abilities (ie, mobility, mental capacity, etc.) are discussed in detail.

This chapter is in large part based on the empirical findings of a recent Swedish study entitled, The Long-Term Care Patient's Immediate Environment.[2] The study involved a screening of the functional status of geriatric patients and their needs for help in activities of daily living (ADL). Based on the findings of the study, guidelines were developed for the design of furniture and other technical equipment so that the independence of the patient in her or his environment could be maximized. The conclusion is that the elderly person's level of functional ability in the immediate environment can be maximized through systematic environmental assessment. The idea of adapting the physical environment to the special needs of the elderly patient can be relevant whether the care is provided in the patient's own home, an acute hospital, or a nursing home. Through systematic assessment of the physical environment, it is possible to design adaptations to meet the special needs of each individual and to give the patient maximal independence and a richer and more meaningful life. Another equally important factor is the way in which adaptations in the living environment can affect the quantity and type of physical labor that is required of the staff. It has been shown that when facilities are adapted to the functional needs of the elderly patient, the staff and patients notice a change in ways in which they interact. When patients are more active and independent and staff have an altered workload and more meaningful personal contact with patients, the mood and motivation of all involved is likely to be more positive and uplifting.

HEALTHY ELDERLY AND THEIR FUNCTIONAL STATUS—WHAT CAN BE EXPECTED?

Physical Abilities

Let us highlight the average functional abilities of the healthy elderly. The older patient, if given a choice, would prefer to recuperate and be rehabilitated while living at home. The elderly have strong ties to their home; thus, the help of the spouse or others (usually older relatives) is crucial to allowing convalescence in their own home. From the beginning, home health care can protect the health of the caregiver and maximize the patient's ability to perform ADL by including a systematic assessment of the living environment as a key part of care planning. Provision of such assistance openly acknowledges that the older caregiver (themselves often in their 80s) has some decrease in physical ability which needs special consideration as it relates to caring for a disabled relative.

It has been demonstrated that >90 percent of persons 75 to 84 years of age can manage without help to perform such tasks as grooming, bathing, dressing, eating, etc.[3] A Swedish study finds that only 3 percent of persons 70 years of age are living in institutions—chronic care or nursing homes.[1] At the age of 79, nine of 10 elderly live in their own home.

Some elderly persons living at home are dependent on nursing care and, when it is provided by another older person, the abilities of the average healthy elderly person must be taken into consideration. Relevant changes in functional abilities noted by Branch and Jette are shown in Table 9-1.

Assessment and adaptation of the physical environment is one way to prevent unnecessary strain on the caregiver, whether an older family member or a nurse's aide. The physical environment is but one aspect of the patient's total environment. The patient's total environment (physical, emotional, and social) is significant; this chapter highlights those changes in the physical environment that help to enrich the patient's possibilities for a meaningful and satisfying lifestyle.

Table 9-1. Change in Functional Abilities

Age (yr)	Can Perform Heavy Housework (%)	Lift Arms Above Shoulder Level (%)	Lift Items Weighing 5 kg (%)	Fine Motor Coordination of Hands (%)
65–74	67	84	82	82
65–74	78	91	96	85
75–84	42	81	67	74
75–84	66	89	90	74

Intellectual Function

The intellect does not deteriorate as dramatically as is often assumed.[1] Actually, for a healthy elderly person, the intellect remains more or less the same from middle age up to 80 years of age. The important difference is that older persons need more time to carry out intellectual functions. Learning to adapt to new environments is more difficult for an elderly person (a strong rationale for home care, when appropriate) and *learning new skills will take longer*. The elderly need reinforcement that learning on this premise (avoiding timed activities) is possible and desirable.

CASE STUDY

Emma is an 80-year-old, alert woman with Parkinson's disease who is actively taking part in what is happening around her at the nursing home in which she is a patient. She is physically very weak. When she lies in her bed, she has no ability to come from a lying position to a seated posture or the reverse. She is unable to sit up without help from the staff. Her inability to sit up independently prevents her from getting an overview of things around her

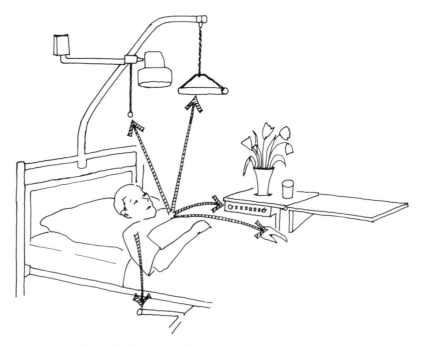

Fig. 9-1.   Patient in bed. Can the patient reach the various levers and controls? [Redrawn from Agranius G, Jäderberg E, Osterman M: Långvårdspatientens närmiljö (The Long-term Care Patient's Immediate Environment). The Swedish Board for Technical Development, Stockholm, 1979.]

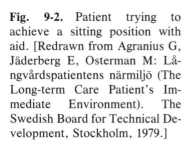

Fig. 9-2. Patient trying to achieve a sitting position with aid. [Redrawn from Agranius G, Jäderberg E, Osterman M: Långvårdspatientens närmiljö (The Long-term Care Patient's Immediate Environment). The Swedish Board for Technical Development, Stockholm, 1979.]

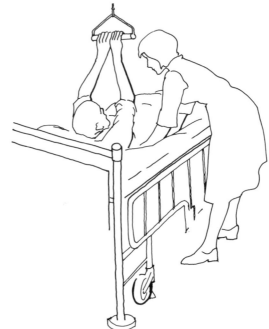

or reaching for something she wants. The controls for adjusting the bed are out of her reach. In addition, if she could reach the levers, they require more strength and dexterity than she has in her hands, forearms, and shoulders. Hence, Emma is totally dependent on staff assistance to achieve a sitting position (Figs. 9-1 and 9-2).

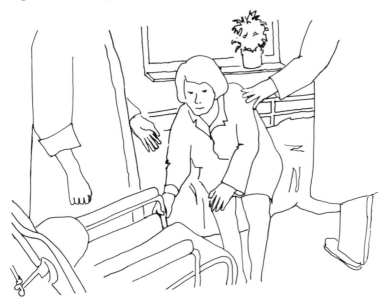

Fig. 9-3.   Transferring from bed to chair.

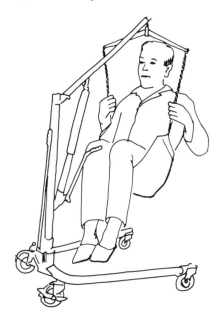

Fig. 9-4. ''Old-fashioned'' lifting device? [Redrawn from Agranius G, Jäderberg E, Osterman M: Långvårdspatientens närmiljö (The Long-term Care Patient's Immediate Environment). The Swedish Board for Technical Development, Stockholm, 1979.]

To transfer from the bed to the wheelchair, Emma requires the help of two nurse's aide. She is barely able to help herself in this ADL. There are no railings on the bed that readily assist her in the transfer to the wheelchair, and the bed and the wheelchair are not compatible pieces of equipment. (That is— the bed and the wheelchair lack the design modifications to allow for ease of use in the desired function of transferring from one to the other Fig. 9-3).

Much of the care Emma requires from the staff is physically strenuous for the staff. Emma is afraid of the equipment that is meant to ease the strain for the staff, since she experiences pain when it is used. The patient experiences the use of some of the equipment as degrading and voices her aversion to the equipment. The result is that the staff is regularly forced to carry out tasks (ADL) in opposition to the wishes of the patient and occasionally with her direct resistance. The equipment often used to lift the patient for shower or bath is continually viewed by the staff and the patient as a problem (Fig. 9-4).

THE IMMEDIATE ENVIRONMENT

The immediate environment for a patient in a hospital or a nursing home room comprises a set of basic furniture: bed, bedside table with instrument panel, bedside lamp, easy chair and/or wheelchair, small chair, table, and cupboard/wardrobe (Fig. 9-5).

Most of the everyday activities for the elderly disabled patient take place in the patient's room. It is also the part of the care environment in which family/staff perform most of the caregiving. Many jobs are carried out around the bed: making the bed; turning; moving up, changing sanitary towels; washing; using

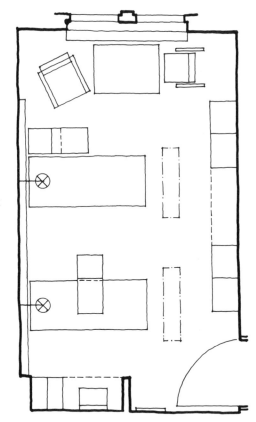

Fig. 9-5. Plan of a typical patient room.

the bedpan; preventing decubiti; assisting the patient in lying down, feeding, dressing; and visits to the toilet, bath, shower, etc. All of these tasks are, to a varying extent, an activity for the patient and a caregiving task for the family/ staff.

When we talk about bed, chair, etc., the concept of furniture is not completely adequate. The functional requirements differ considerably from what we find in an ordinary home environment. It may be more relevant to use the term technical equipment. This does not imply that technical equipment and a homelike atmosphere cannot be combined. Achievement of this atmosphere, however, requires a different approach to design than that which has given us the standard nursing home equipment and furniture of today.

Furniture/technical equipment must be designed based on the functions of an average healthy elderly person. To a certain extent, these standardized units should be adaptable to the requirements and capacities of different patients. A range of factors must be considered in designing furniture adequate to the needs of the elderly.

1. Muscle strength and joint mobility are greatly decreased in long-term

care patients. This causes considerable deterioration in the function of arms and hands and influences patients' ability to use the equipment.

2. The range of reaching decreases with increasing age, and it is *not* realistic to expect an old patient to reach out a distance >50 cm, lift arms above 70° flexion and 45° abduction, perform full extension of the elbow joint, or have considerable external rotation at the shoulder.

3. This group of patients commonly can use only one arm, the function of which is reduced. A two-handed grasp should therefore not be required.

4. Many elderly patients have distinct difficulties in utilizing the information that is required to manage combined movements (2 or 3 stage commands). Such movements therefore should not be required in order to move and use equipment or furniture.

5. Great fluctuations in the patient's physical and mental capacity can be anticipated due to variations in medical illness and motivation. These variations must be compensated for by the flexibility of the equipment.

6. Dizziness and problems with balance in combination with mobility problems mean that the long-term-care patient must be able to trust the immediate environment. Patients need suitably placed *"fixed-points"* to pull themselves up, as well as provide the ability to shift the burden of body weight, when this is no longer within the patients' voluntary capacity. This requires that the equipment offer suitable grasp possibilities and that it not roll away or tip over when patients lean on it.

EMPIRICAL EXPERIMENTS

The above analysis of the immediate environment is based on a project done for the Swedish Board for Technical Development (STU).[2] The project has been described in detail,[2] and the information presented here is drawn from that study.

The project involved a screening of geriatric patients living in nursing homes and specifically observed their functional status and need for help and support in ADL. The results have provided a basis for design standards and functional descriptions of the immediate environment in addition to increased knowledge about efficient work routines for nursing care and rehabilitation, use of space, etc.

So that the ways in which the patient's needs and capabilities were fulfilled in a certain environment could be studied, the patients were divided into "needs groups" based on their physical and mental status, which was mirrored by their need for assistance with ADL. To define the groups, ADL were categorized according to their levels of difficulty.

Patients were placed in needs groups based on actual ability to perform independently the tasks listed. The categorization of functional activities was developed from the perspective of the patients (Table 9-2).

Table 9-2. Needs Groups

Needs Group	Definition	Patient Activity/Need
No expressed needs	Patients lack the capacity to make active demands on their environment	All care is provided by the staff to the patient
Basic functional needs	Patients needs are of a basic nature and can be satisfied if the patients' state of health allows it	Changes from sitting-lying position; summons assistance; drinks without help, and switches on light
Personal requirements	Patients have needs concerning simple activities of daily living that are important for the preservation of their self-esteem	Needs to have access to important belongings; to read, write, listen, and be able to move about room and to eat a meal; attends to basic hygiene and goes to the toilet, if necessary with assistance
Activity requirements	Patients require activities that maintain and develop their capacity for exterior activities	Independently mobile; attends to hygiene; needs work/meaningful activity and to attend to personal belongings

Group 1

Group 1 comprised patients with no active physical abilities. The patients in this group had a total need for help for all ADL. The design of the environment is of vital importance for the workload of the nursing staff.

Group 2

Group 2 comprised patients with basic needs. The patients in this group had a very restricted physical and/or mental ability. The activities defined as relevant to this group were:

To change body posture
To call for attention/help
To turn on a lamp
To drink

The organization of the patients environment that is within arm's reach is crucial to maximizing patient participation. All heavy tasks are carried out by the staff, and the design of the environment is thus very important to them as well.

Group 3

Group 3 comprised patients with personal needs. These patients had the ability to carry out many ADL that are important to one's sense of independence and self-respect. The activities relevant to this group were:

To eat a meal
To have access to personal belongings
To read, write, and listen
To wash hands, face, etc.
To go to the toilet (with help if needed)
To have a little mobility (walking or in a wheelchair)

The design of the environment is of equal importance to staff and patient.

Group 4

Group 4 comprised patients with active needs. The patients had a pronounced wish to carry out most day-to-day activities in order to develop or keep their mental ability, physical strength, and self-esteem. The additional activities relevant to this group were:

To have independent mobility in the room
To work or to perform personally fulfilling activities and to have a sense of belonging
To take care of personal belongings
To take responsibility for personal hygiene
To use the toilet

The design of the environment is of vital importance, in order to maximize the patients' functional ability.

Measurements of the patients' movement capacity, hand strength, and reach to equipment were made. The sample of patients was chosen to be representative of the typical distribution of patients at a long-term facility.

The results showed that > 80 percent of the patients were capable of carrying out ADL as defined for groups 3 and 4, *but only* if the immediate environment was adapted to their needs. The detailed experiments with patients trying to perform different activities showed that a badly designed environment made it practically impossible for the patient to carry out ADL (Figs. 9-6 and 9-7).

The most common problems were related to:

1. The equipment itself, (ie, controls and grips are out of arm's reach).
2. The lack of means for the patient to adjust between a lying and a seated posture in order to get an overview of personal possessions or to reach them.
3. The fact that the strength needed to use equipment/furniture was more than the patient possessed, and/or handling demanded two hands.
4. Badly designed grips, if any.
5. Coordination between different pieces of equipment:
    a. Bed table did not function safely/effectively together with beds and

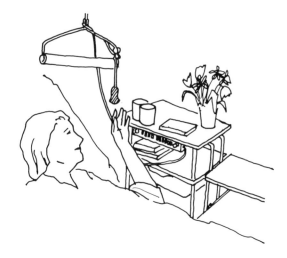

Fig. 9-6. Difficulties in reaching the alarm/call button. [Redrawn from Agranius G, Jäderberg E, Osterman M: Långvårdspatientens närmiljö (The Long-term Care Patient's Immediate Environment). The Swedish Board for Technical Development, Stockholm, 1979.]

chairs; it could not be put in the best position for use, and the drawers could not be opened down and thereby positioned within reach.

b. Chairs and wheelchairs worked badly together with the bed.

6. Space available:

a. Different pieces of equipment could not be put in the best position in relation to each other or to the patient.

b. A patient in a wheelchair was "shut out" from parts of the room's perceptual demands.

7. The patient's lack of understanding of working of controls and/or ability to differentiate between the different controls and symbols.

The empirical observations described point out that Emma may use much of her energy on meaningless and unnecessary tasks such as using various tricks to try to reach the lamp or to try to get over to the wheelchair. For many patients, the route from the bed to the bathroom is filled with tiresome obsta-

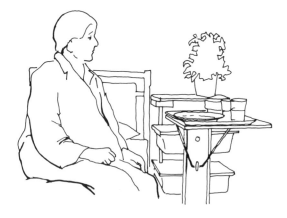

Fig. 9-7. Ineffective sitting posture for eating. [Redrawn from Agranius G, Jäderberg E, Osterman M: Långvårdspatientens närmiljö (The Long-term Care Patient's Immediate Environment). The Swedish Board for Technical Development, Stockholm, 1979.]

cles. Often, patients who manage to perform the desired task have no energy left for more stimulating activities. The staff may also be inclined to speed up the process by helping more than is necessary. Hence, the patient loses both skills and self-confidence.

The Swedish study[2] was followed by experiments in which guidelines for improvements and new design principles were tested.[4,5] The purpose was to enhance the patient's control over the immediate environment and to increase the patient's potential for maximal independence in self-care and meaningful activities.

BED

The bed is probably the most important piece of furniture, especially for the elderly person who is bound to spend long periods of time in bed not only at night but also during the day. Most beds are constructed in a way that makes it very difficult for a weak and old person to perform even simple tasks such as changing body position, adjusting the backrest, or reaching a glass in order to drink. The possible sitting positions are as a rule very uncomfortable. Tests undertaken with the help of bedridden elderly patients showed that their ability to adjust their posture played a crucial role. When they could find a comfortable and functional position, they felt better and were able to reach things they needed in their immediate environment. The design of the backrest and the sitting area of the bed is very important, as are the dimensions of the bed as compared with body measurements, and the positioning of the backrests. These factors strongly influence the ability of a person to cope without assistance from the staff (Fig. 9-8).

Extensive experiments with different types of railings and supports show that their appropriate placement plays a key role in improving patients' mobility. With the use of appropriate railings, all elderly patients tested showed an improved ability to get in and out of bed. Patients who were normally de-

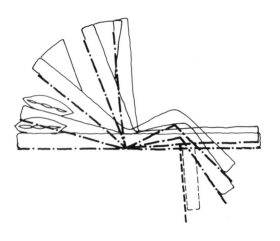

Fig. 9-8. Design of bed with adjustable bottom. [Redrawn from Jaderberg E, Karlqvist L, Kube E: Säng och Sängbudna Aktiviteter (The Bed and Bedridden Activities). The Swedish Board for Technical Development Stockholm, 1982.]

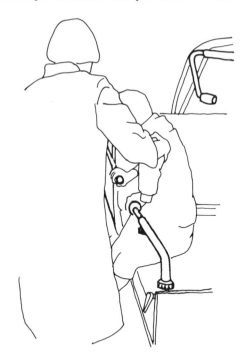

Fig. 9-9. Rails for changing body position and allowing ease of transferring. [Redrawn from Jaderberg E, Karlqvist L, Kube E: Säng och Sängbudna Aktiviteter (The Bed and Bedridden Activities). The Swedish Board for Technical Development Stockholm, 1982.]

pendent on total help from the staff could now get from the bed to the wheelchair with the assistance of only one person (Fig. 9-9). Railings are an essential part of the equipment around the patient's bed. Other improvements can be made by a careful placement of furniture and equipment in the immediate environment.

The amount of light also plays a crucial role in maximizing functional abilities for the elderly patient. Six important elements of the environment should be within arms reach of the bed.

Backrest

The angle of the bed's backrest determines the ability of the patient to reach, to see and get an overview, to achieve a suitable position for various activities, and to be able to change body position in order not to become unnecessarily tired. A backrest that can truly be controlled by the patient is a must.

Alarm

All patients must be able to reach an alarm or call button. The alarm should have a fixed place and, in addition, there should be a flexible device that can be adjusted and placed according to the individual needs of a patient. It should be easily distinguishable from other controls, easy to use, give a feedback to the patient to confirm that the signal for help has been activated; it should not cause false alarms or be a risk or an obstacle for the patient. The flexible unit should be cordless.

Bed Light

Most activities demand good light. This demand increases with age. The lamp should be placed within comfortable reach. The direction of the light should be changeable. The switch should be placed on or close to the lamp and should be well defined; the intensity of light should be controlled by the same switch.

Radio and Television

The controls for radio and television should be within normal reach of the patient. Soft headsets should be available within normal reach.

Work Surface

To allow the patient the best possibility of eating, drinking, and reading, etc., without too much assistance, a work surface must be within reach (the patient's reach). It should be big enough (approximately the width of the bed times the length of the underarm). The height of the work space/table should be adjustable. The surface of the work space should be textured (provide friction) so that objects placed on the surface do not slide. The surface should be sturdy and stable so that the patient can lean against it and, when necessary, derive support for the arms. The patient should be able to push it away and pull it into a comfortable position. To allow the patient to read, a support is needed against which the book or paper can rest. It should be possible to adjust the height and inclinations of the book support without changing the distance from the eye (Fig. 9-10).

Chair

Earlier studies showed that the "chair" is traditionally a weak part of the elderly patient's environment. The chairs on the market can, only to a very limited extent, fulfill the functional requirements of a disabled person. Patients who are bound to spend their time and perform most of their activities seated have different needs than do those who are mobile and live at home and/or use the open care system. The gap between functional demands and existing sitting

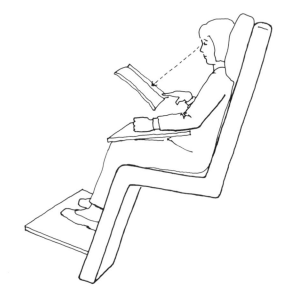

Fig. 9-10. Bed adjusted for reading. [Redrawn from Jaderberg E, Karlqvist L, Kube E: Säng och Sängbudna Aktiviteter (The Bed and Bedridden Activities). The Swedish Board for Technical Development Stockholm, 1982.]

furniture increases stress on patients and staff, especially when lifting and moving the patient is necessary.

Our investigations and experiments show that several types of chairs are needed to meet the demands from patients and staff. The traditional wheelchair is essentially a means of transportation. It is well suited for long or fast transports (eg, to external activities outside the ward); however, for the chair-ridden patient, this aspect plays a minor role. The overriding function for many disabled elderly is the sitting function. It is essential that the various types of chairs, with the possible exception of transportation chairs, optimize the sitting function. The patient should be able to sit comfortably and to take the sitting posture best suited for the activity at hand. The staff should be able to work with the patient and the chair without unnecessary strain.

The starting point is what we term the "comfort chair," a chair in which it is comfortable to sit. According to the patient's activity level, self-control, or needs for assistance, other functions are added to the chair, such as a means to get in and out of the chair or a means of mobility. There is need for a chair that can be used for "work," especially in small and narrow spaces such as around the bed or in the bathroom or shower area. To solve the problem of sitting, it is essential to make it possible for the patient to change from one type of chair to another when necessary. The transfer function is of great importance. To fulfill all the demands from stationary sitting to transportation, a whole range of chairs would be needed—from a comfortable armchair to chairs with wheels and lifting and transportation functions, to the traditional wheelchair for long-distance transportation of the patient.

People who work with patients feel that it is difficult to introduce more chairs. The space in the patient's room is limited. The number of chairs need not increase. Today, two types of chairs are found in most facilities. The traditional armchair, which is often difficult for a disabled patient to use, and the standard wheelchair, which is brought in to solve acute problems. In the future, these traditional types of chairs should be *replaced* by comfort chairs with a good sitting function and equipped with devices to effect transferring movements and transportation according to the patient's needs; if necessary, it should be supplemented by a special transportation chair.

It is not possible to discuss here the design criteria and the highly exacting requirements that must be imposed on the chair. The present generation of chairs used in the care system has weaknesses. There is a need for better:

Adjustments of position of the chair for different activities.

Adjustment within certain dimensions of the chair, according to the size of the patient's trunk, arms, legs, etc., and the disease of the patient.

System design, through which the chairs function together with other equipment. Each unit should fulfill (apart from its primary function) its function related to transferring, thereby allowing the patient easy egress as well as access. (see Chapter 6)

SOME CONCLUDING REMARKS

At times it is argued that an environment well adapted to the needs of the elderly patient can be a threat to the relations between patient and staff, and that this is an excuse for the management to save on personnel costs. This argument reflects an outmoded view of what care is all about. The modern attitude, expressed in a recent Swedish report on local nursing homes[6] emphasizes that:

> the accomplishments of the care team should primarily aim at *supporting* and *activating* the patient, so that she can manage her daily tasks independently to the largest possible extent" [italics added]

and

> a well planned physical environment is a precondition for the patient to participate to his/her fullest capacity and to allow the staff to help in a way that is safe and effective for both the patient and the staff members. The physical environment should make it easier for the patient to be active in spite of functional disabilities and the staff should be offered a good working-environment.

Many of the patients at ordinary hospitals are >65 years of age. The elderly patients also spend the longest time at the hospital. Every third patient on the medical wards in Stockholm hospitals is waiting for a bed at some other institution. The waiting time is often perceived as trying by the staff, since they regard the patient as a closed case. If the time in the hospital were used to regain and/or maintain the patient's functional skills/motivation, it would be of great value, especially for the personnel who will care for the patient later. A well-organized immediate environment can facilitate a patient's ability and sense of well-being. A well-adapted environment is important to the ability of elderly and handicapped persons who are living in their own homes to remain in an old, familiar environment. For personnel, it is essential to support the home environment with proper equipment, organized in a meaningful way. New furniture and technical equipment cost money. In the long run, however, the potential gains of a well-adapted immediate environment are considerable. The care of elderly and disabled patients is a demanding task. It takes a heavy toll in terms of a high staff turnover and many health problems among the staff. With more active, independent patients and easier and more rewarding patient contact for the staff, the quality of care will increase. Costs will be favorably affected. The big return for a well-adapted environment, however, will be not only money but the possibility of offering the patient a richer life with increased self-respect and personal integrity.

REFERENCES

1. William-Olsson M, Svanborg A: Gammal eller ung på äldre dar (young or old in older days). Utbildningsproduktion, Malmö, 1984
2. Agranius G, Jäderberg E, Österman M: Långvårdspatientens närmiljö (The Long-Term Care Patient's Immediate Environment). The Swedish Board for Technical Development, Stockholm, 1979
3. Branch L, Jette A: The Framingham Disability Study: Social Disability among the Aging. Am J Public Health 71:1202, 1981
4. Jäderberg E, Karlqvist L, Kube E: Säng och Sängbundna Aktiviteter (The Bed and Bedridden Activities). The Swedish board for Technical Development, Stockholm, 1981
5. Karlqvist L, Kube E, Söderström C, Österman M: Stol och Stolsbundna Aktiviteter (The Chair and Chairridden Activities). The Swedish Board for Technical Development, Stockholm, 1982
6. Loklala sjukhem (Local Nursing Homes). SPRI, Stockholm, 1979

10 | Ethical Considerations

Ruth B. Purtilo

If United States Census Bureau predictions are correct, by the year 2025 more than 55 million Americans will be 65 years of age.[1] Almost every source predicts that the disproportionately large percentage of the nation's health care monies expended on the elderly population will continue to increase with their increasing numbers. Therefore, today more urgently than ever, solid ethical guidelines are needed in order to assure that the elderly population—a large and potentially disenfranchised group—will be treated in a manner that is morally justifiable.

No special ethical principles are required for assessing the moral dilemmas raised by health care for elderly patients.[2] The guidelines in ethical codes and such principles as "do no harm," and "the patient's rights to life and autonomy" apply to all groups of patients. However, an elderly person may have special needs and values that will give rise to a somewhat different judgment about what ought to be done in a treatment decision. Some ethical concerns that often arise in the treatment interventions of elderly patients will be addressed in this chapter under the following headings: (1) respect for the person, (2) autonomy and informed consent, and (3) justice-related issues. As each is addressed, the reader can begin to understand better how special needs and values of the elderly patient become factors as physical therapists attempt to make ethically supportable treatment decisions.

RESPECT FOR THE PERSON

Principle I of the American Physical Therapy Association Code of Ethics states that the physical therapist must respect the rights and dignity of all individuals.[3] Almost everyone would interpret such a statement to mean that an individual's unique needs, desires, fears, and hopes must be taken into account when an intervention is being contemplated. To do less is to treat the person as less than human or, as Kant declared, to treat a person as a means rather than as an end. In so doing, the duty "not to harm" clearly is compromised.

Difficulty in perceiving the elderly person as a unique individual often prevents the most well-intentioned health professional from respecting the patient's dignity. One reason for this moral "blind spot" is the difficulty of projecting one's imagination across the years to imagine what it is like to be old. Another reason is that the elderly population has emerged as a distinct societal group, complete with stereotyped assumptions about how old people think and act. Whenever a group of shared characteristics can be designated by one stereotypical term, the group has been *labeled*. How does the label of "the elderly" influence the health professional's intent to treat the patient as an individual?

Labels are highly instrumental tools in communication. Without them, every description would become bogged down in detail. For instance, most persons >65 years of age become grouped as "elderly" for purposes of efficiently enabling procedures related to insurance, vital statistics, retirement requirements, and human service privileges. But although the label clearly allows efficiency within a bureaucratic society, individuals initially respond to the designation with varying degrees of denial, embarrassment, horror, or resignation. In spite of their response, as years go by, the label becomes more indelible. As one 85-year-old woman suffering from severe rheumatoid arthritis told me, "Some days the aches are less, and I feel young again," then I look in the mirror and I see this (she pointed to her very wrinkled face). No one sees me as anything but 'elderly'." The tenacity of old age, which forces persons to be labeled as one of "the aged" or "the elderly," persists like the chirping of a cricket on a warm night. Modern society demands that older individuals largely be forever recognized, reasoned about, and reckoned with as a *group*, blurring individual differences. Health professionals, as much as anyone else, must continually fight against the images of the elderly that would make it impossible to view an individual elderly patient as different in any regard from the rest of "the elderly."

On a positive note, a well-defined notion of "the elderly" or "aged" can foster ideas and adaptations leading to better care of older persons. For example, a medical student recently wrote:

> I will work with the elderly, not always hoping for cure, but always working for stability in illness and a quality of life that lends meaning to those who have already lived so long.[4]

This health professional is among a growing number who reject a narrowly conceived mandate of health care limited to acute interventions only, understanding that in health care one must "cure sometimes, comfort always." Such an orientation is badly needed in developing a realistic approach to treatment of individual elderly patients, some of whom are more physically and mentally capable than others. Recently the *Journal of Rehabilitation*[5] devoted an entire issue to the rehabilitation of older persons, building a strong case for more programs, better demographic information to highlight differences among individuals, and improved skills and understanding of an old persons' individual needs. The Center for Demographic Studies at Duke University has invested enormous energy in evaluating concepts of morbidity and mortality in the elderly, its goal being to reflect more accurately individual differences in need and capability among members of this group.[6] These examples help to highlight the ways in which (once the label of "elderly" was implemented) the identification of a *group* needing attention actually served to foster policies and practices among health professionals that respect elderly patients as *individuals*.

However, here another caveat is needed. Identification of need per se is an insufficient criterion for assuring that a group will receive high-quality treatment. The treatment of European Jews during the Nazi years is a grisly reminder that identification and labeling of a group's supposed characteristics by no means assures that attentiveness to the special needs of individuals in the group will follow. In an "ageist" society that clearly values youth, able-bodied persons, and independence, an indelible label applied to older persons places them in an extremely vulnerable position as a group *and* as individuals.

Even among health professionals who believe themselves sympathetic to the needs of an elderly patient, prejudicial ageist attitudes can creep into clinical judgment. For example, an article entitled "Stroke in the Geriatric Patient" largely is sympathetic to the special problems of treating older persons who have had strokes. However, the author states, "for the elderly person surviving a completed stroke, who cannot benefit from many of the usual interventions, the prognosis is often not dire." The author makes this judgment on the following basis: "While there is high frequency of occupational disability following stroke, most patients in the group we are considering are already retired."[7] The statement, which may not seem problematic superficially, suggests that older stroke patients do not need *work* skills. But what of those who still actively engage in an occupation? And which of the skills would not also be critically important for the accomplishment of other aspects of daily living for elderly persons who no longer are employed in the labor force?

Finally, the label, "elderly," must be viewed as a double-edged sword whose swath can cut opportunity or destruction for individuals in the group. Health care practices directed toward this group will be determined largely by the decisions of health professionals who have made a commitment to working with this group and by policy-makers. Being guided by the dictum, "Do no harm," the alterations, innovations, and creations of health professionals engaged in geriatric health care must reflect individual needs, desires, and hopes. Each health professional must try to sort out the effect of the stereotypes embodied in the labeling of the elderly when making a treatment decision about an elderly individual. Without continual discernment along these lines, the health professional becomes vulnerable to treating the patient with less than the full human respect he or she deserves.

AUTONOMY AND INFORMED CONSENT

A common criticism of modern health care is the health professional's inability or unwillingness to make patients more fully involved in their own treatment. Many of these criticisms rest on the patient's right to autonomy. The idea of autonomy suggests that it is morally necessary to allow individuals to act in a way consistent with their own desires and needs. Limits on autonomy are usually set at those boundaries where a person's behavior becomes self-destructive, foolish, or tragic. The idea of a patient as an autonomous agent serves to place an obligation on health professionals to respect the values of the patient and not to let their own values unduly influence decisions about treatment. The conflict between the two sets of values becomes perhaps the most troublesome when a patient refuses life-saving treatment when the health professional believes that the patient should be treated. However, even in that difficult circumstance, the decision of a competent patient must be respected in most cases.[8] Some philosophers go so far today as to insist that the concept of a person as an autonomous agent is central to all further understanding of persons.

The health professional who is treating an elderly patient is faced with a significant challenge in trying to assure that the patient's autonomy is being protected. Most elderly people already have lost autonomy in some other area of their life. Age-related dependence arising from the social, physical, and intellectual effects of aging and/or illness necessitates the assistance of others for many elderly people in aspects of life in which they formerly exercised self-determination. Exacerbating the deleterious effects of these types of dependence are role expectations and norms adopted by some older people because they believe them appropriate for someone of their age. For instance, one study showed that in regard to an elderly patient's participation in a clinical research project, the members of the group seemed to be *most* influenced by the expectations of those around them and by what they saw their *peers* doing.[9] Clearly, the learned role expectations and norms were instrumental in their decision about what to do.

The dependence on family members probably also influences many older persons' decisions about what to do when faced with a decision. A study distributed to 37 adults aged 50 to 96 years asked the subjects to describe a moral problem they faced in daily life and what attempts were made to try to resolve it. In the "old" old group (>71 years of age), most of the moral conflict focused on the relationship of the subject with a family member. The primary goal of the respondent was a desire to maintain a harmonious interpersonal relationship with that person.[10] This study suggests that the decision of an older person to follow a course of action may be highly influenced by a need to maintain a harmonious relationship, often within a situation in which the patient is dependent. Therefore, the older patient whose opinion is sought about a course of treatment may understandably be relying very heavily on what he or she believes the family member or significant other(s) will accept.

The health professional working with the elderly patient often is tempted to help the patient make a "better" choice by becoming very directive with the patient. Often the intent is to help the patient make a considered choice, although it has the effect of further diminishing the patient's autonomy. Dworkin, who has written widely in the area of autonomy, maintains that paternalism, the practice of intervening to help the patient make a decision, is permissible if it "preserves and enhances for the individual his ability rationally to consider and carry out his own decisions."[11] This kind of paternalism may be acceptable in that it places elderly persons in a protected "milieu" of autonomy:

> a milieu over which they may then exercise as much control as is consistent with the (health professional's) objective assessment of their deficits and their subjective perception of their benefits, not vice versa.[12]

The mechanism of informed consent has been developed to help patients to express their autonomy more fully and to foster much-needed trust between health professional and patient. As described in more detail elsewhere, I believe that the minimum information that should be included as a part of the interaction designed to enable a patient to make an informed decision about physical therapy intervention includes:

1. A description of the patients' current status as it relates to the perceived need for physical therapy services.
2. A description of the assessment procedure(s) or intervention(s) of choice indicated for clarifying the condition or treating it, as well as alternative procedures or interventions.
3. A list of the risks and benefits of the procedures and interventions as far as the physical therapist can judge them.
4. Additional information that the physical therapist believes will assist a particular patient in arriving at an informed choice.
5. An offer to answer questions later as they arise.
6. Any additional information recommended by policies or legal counsel of the institution.[13]

A patient who gives informed consent is involved in problem solving. Very often, problem-solving ability changes with age. In old age, the memory may get slower, and the problem to be solved may be defined differently; the relation of the problem to former problems faced by the patient, and the organization of the various parts of the problem may differ.[14] Although this does not indicate that the patient necessarily has *worse* problem-solving ability, it very much supports the idea that the health professional must take into account the possibility that the elderly patient's perceptions and abilities have changed and that adaptations in the language/communication style may be necessary.

Of central concern in the issue of informed consent is the notion of competence. Because consent cannot be informed if the client is not competent to make a decision about the proposed treatment, competence becomes a governing factor in trying to decide how to proceed.

Competence can be established on several levels. Fromer illustrates:

> [A] person of limited intelligence may be considered legally incompetent though he is perfectly able to conduct his personal affairs, maintain a home, and hold a job. If he were to enter a hospital, he might be considered incompetent to sign a consent form, which is a legal document, though he may understand ramifications of the procedure if it is explained in language at his level of comprehension. Sometimes the level of competence varies over time; a person may be competent to decide a matter today that he may not be able to decide in the future if his life situation changes.[15]

Because competence varies from time to time and in differing situations, some authors have proposed the idea of intermittent or "limited" competence. This would preclude someone's being determined either totally competent or totally incompetent, preserving as much autonomy as possible.[16] These concepts are especially relevant to the elderly patient who is afflicted with "sundown syndrome" (a state in which normal mental abilities are operant during the day but decrease drastically in function at night).

In summary, the patient's right to autonomy should be a governing factor in deciding a course of treatment intervention. Informed consent is a mechanism designed to assure and enhance autonomy. The individual's needs and values must be taken into account in this process. Assuring the highest degree possible of self-determination for the elderly patient is a challenge that must be met by the health professional if high quality care is the goal.

JUSTICE-RELATED ISSUES

A discussion of ethical issues regarding treatment interventions for elderly persons would be incomplete without mention of justice-related considerations in health care. The author of an article entitled, Will The First Medicare Generation Be The Last? is pessimistic about the viability of the present treatment plan for elderly persons, seeing it as a benefit for "a privileged special interest group." Rather than viewing it as a first step toward comprehensive insurance coverage for all Americans, he views Medicare as an "unwarranted and overgenerous public program for those whose needs seem to dictate no such special attention."[17]

Although generally critical of the program, the emphasis in this commentor's remarks is that the Medicare provision should serve the elderly who can show *financial* need rather than allot care on the basis of *medical* need. Such a program would still rest on a *need* criterion, and the allocations themselves would flow from a "needs-based" understanding of distributive justice.

Distributive justice considerations directly affect many policies and practices. The goal of distributive justice is limitation of arbitrary distinctions among individuals or groups, thereby assuring a proper share to each party who has legitimate claim to the thing that is being distributed (eg, health care services). Therefore, although justice is not the only value related to assuring a humane system of health care toward the elderly, it is certainly an important one.[18]

Three commonly accepted criteria for allocating a society's resources are (1) special merits of some persons, (2) the ability of some to make a greater societal contribution than others, and (3) the special needs of some persons. Clearly, the commentator on Medicare sees the needs approach as the most equitable approach to health care resources, although he would add to it the idea of *financial* need. A principle of allocation based on need entails the idea that society has an obligation to take care of its members and that persons unable to meet their own basic needs are entitled to resources. The governing question becomes one of methods of assuring funds for so vital a dimension of social well-being.

Any health professional practicing today knows that grave concern is being voiced about the effects of an increased number of elderly patients who will consume an ever-expanding amount of health care services. Cost–benefit and cost-effectiveness analyses have been used to provide quantitative methods for guiding the allocation of health care resources. These approaches attempt to give specific numerical values to the benefits and costs of medical interventions of various kinds. Avorn, of the Division on Aging at Harvard Medical School, shows persuasively that cost–benefit and cost-efficiency approaches to health policy for the elderly are fraught with difficulty. At best, it is impossible to account for all of the costs and benefits that are important in the understanding of health care for this group. At worst, these approaches are a method of "turning age discrimination into health policy." He points out, for instance, that the "unproductivity" of many elderly is, ironically, a double jeopardy, since mandatory retirement often forces elderly workers out of the workplace—elderly workers who are then valued less because they are "unproductive."[19]

Almost anyone reading the literature on the long-term implications of Diagnostic Related Groups, (DRGs), is forced to conclude that those most hurt by the present arrangements will be the DRG population, >65 years of age. DRGs are compelling institutions to be more fully influenced by the economics of care than ever before; the institutions thus will increasingly be forced to discontinue treatment prematurely for elderly persons with long-term illnesses. The emphasis on a legitimate worry about the increasing costs of health care has allowed some practitioners boldly to suggest health care policies clearly not in the best interests of large numbers of people (eg, the elderly). For example, a recent article in a leading medical journal suggests that not only is there no longer a strong claim on the health professions to provide long-term care within hospitals, but also that in recent medical history there never was.[20]

These events place the health professional in a position of being compromised in regards to his or her best judgment regarding the health care needed for elderly patients. A health professional who is unwilling to become involved in health policy formation and evaluation increasingly will be frustrated by being unable to offer quality (or any) treatment interventions. Although the emphasis on not overtreating has been prevalent in the writings of the last decade, the coming decade may well include an equal number of pleas for continuing treatment to a reasonable degree for those with conditions that are not regarded as legitimate foci of attention in the allocation of health care resources. The requirement for health professionals to engage at the level of health policy will be unpalatable to many who do not like to get into the "dirty work" of politics and government. Nonetheless, no greater challenge faces the health professional in the treatment of the elderly than that of becoming a voice for the all-too-often voiceless, assuring a fair allocation of health care resources.

CONCLUDING COMMENT

The above discussion by no means exhausts the wealth of material that could be produced in regard to ethical issues involved in the treatment of an elderly patient. The attempt has been to highlight three major themes that are important in a general assessment of the topic. This chapter should remind the physical therapist of some of the needs and values that the elderly person brings to the treatment situation. The health professional who is guided by the code of ethics and who is mindful of the long-standing moral principle of doing no harm and of the patient's right to autonomy is in a strong position to proceed in a manner that affirms the patient as a person.

REFERENCES

1. United States Bureau of the Census. Current Population Reports Series P25 No. 704, 1977
2. Young EWD: Health care and research in the aged. I. p. 68. In Reich WT (ed): Encyclopedia of Bioethics. Free Press, New York, 1978
3. American Physical Therapy Association Code of Ethics. American Physical Therapy Association, Alexandria, Virginia
4. Kynoff L: Geriatrician: in spite of. p. 14. In Winning Essays: Human Values in the Health Care of the Elderly. Society for Health and Human Values, Philadelphia, 1978
5. Bozarth JO: The rehabilitation process and older people. J Rehabil 47:28, 1981
6. Manton KG: Changing concepts of morbidity and mortality in the elderly population. Milbank Mem Fund Q 60:182, 1982
7. Robbins S: Stroke in the geriatric patient. Hosp Pract 2:293, 1976
8. Miller BL: Autonomy and the refusal of lifesaving therapy. Hastings Center Report 12:4:7, 1981
9. Brody EM: Environmental factors in dependency. p. 81. In Exton-Smith AN, Evans JG (eds): In Care of the Elderly: Meeting the Challenge of Dependency. Grune & Stratton, Orlando, Fla, 1977
10. Rybash JM, Roodin PA, Hoyer WJ: Expressions of moral thought in later adulthood. Gerontologist 23:254, 1983
11. Dworkin G: Paternalism. Monist 56:64, 1972

12. Ratzan R: Being old makes you different: the elderly as research subjects. Hastings Center Report 10:2:32, 1980

13. Purtilo R: Applying the principles of informed consent to patient care: legal and ethical considerations for physical therapy. Phys Ther 64:934, 1984

14. Birren JE: Age and decision strategies. p. 23. In Welford AT, Birren JE (eds): Decision-Making and Age: Interdisciplinary Topics in Gerontology. Karger, New York, 1969

15. Fromer MJ: Ethical Issues in Health Care. CV Mosby, St. Louis, 1981

16. Beauchamp TL, Childress J: The principles of autonomy. p. 69. Principles of Biomedical Ethics. Oxford University Press, New York 1979

17. Bayer R: Will the first medicare generation be the last? Hastings Center Report 14:3:17, 1984

18. Purtilo RB: Social justice in chronic illness and long-term care. p. 371. In Cassel C. Walsh J (eds): Geriatric Medicine: Principles and Practice, II. Springer, New York, 1984

19. Avorn J: Benefit and cost analysis in geriatric care: turning age discrimination into health policy. N Engl J Med 310:1294, 1984

20. Gillick MR: Is the care of the chronically ill a medical prerogative? N Engl J Med 310:190, 1984

11 | The Bobath Approach and the Geriatric Stroke Patient

Isabelle Bohman

The neurodevelopmental treatment (NDT) (Bobath) approach to adult hemiplegic patients, regardless of age, encompasses management of the whole person, emotionally and physically, helping patients to relearn management of their own bodies again. The emphasis is on achieving a better quality of life through functioning with a better quality of movement, one that is more efficient, easier, and thus more pleasurable. This is particularly important for the older person whose physical status may already have been compromised. Age alone is not the determining factor for rehabilitation. Many factors interact and must be considered, but even improved bed mobility without contractures or independence in a wheelchair is a worthwhile goal. One should strive for the highest possible level of safe independence.

As the average person ages, even without hemiplegia, he or she tends to move less; this can lead to disuse atrophy and a general loss of mobility in trunk, neck, and limbs. There may also be arthritis with pain on movement. Diseases may develop, resulting in circulatory problems, and heart rate and respiration become reduced. It becomes a vicious cycle. The lack of mobility may result partially from the lack of power and extension against gravity. Movement against gravity is an effort, and maintaining of erect posture against gravity is even more difficult. Added to these problems is the lack of balance, partially due to lack of trunk mobility and stability. As a result of poor balance the person moves less, fearful of falling, and also stiffens the whole body against falling, especially the limbs. Reduced proprioceptive information and the lack

183

of feeling one's body contributes to decreased balance and may be reinforced by problems of vision, or loss of hearing.

The geriatric patient with hemiplegia has the same problems *plus* asymmetry and abnormal postural tone, either high or low, which interfere with movement of the head, trunk, and limbs. The NDT (Bobath) approach often begins by affording the patient more mobility in the trunk, both upper and lower, and then helping the patient become more symmetrical by learning to use the muscles of the trunk more equally and to control the increased range of movement against gravity. A mobile as well as a stable base (ie, the trunk) allows for better balance in the trunk and greatly assists in regaining easier and better use of the limbs. Better trunk mobility and control also help improve oral–motor function, respiration, and most other vital functions, which in turn has a very positive influence on the person's emotional state and sense of well-being. Obtaining stability with mobility in the postural control of the trunk is key to providing a more symmetrical and functional base from which the head and limbs can function. The patient then relearns normal coordination of head, trunk, and limb movement.

To be functionally independent, a person must achieve the ability to stabilize and move in several postures, ie, horizontal (supine and side-lying) and vertical (sitting and standing). As soon as some control of these postures occurs, the person should assist in moving in and out of these postures, primarily using head and trunk movements but also the limbs to assist balance and to provide support during the transition, eg, supine to side-lying, supine to sitting, or sitting to standing. If one relates posture to function, the essential postures are vertical, ie, sitting and standing and the ability to move between them while controlling the body against gravity. In the vertical postures, the person uses the limbs in weight-bearing to help achieve control of the posture by increasing the base of support. Once better control in the trunk is achieved, the person begins using one or both limbs in functions such as walking or manipulation of tools for upper limb activity. Control of a posture, although not complete balance, always precedes moving in and out of postures or functioning in that posture. This principle is true developmentally but is also applicable when one is working with elderly hemiplegia patients. It is important to work both in sitting and standing postures as soon as possible to help the patient achieve control of the alignment of head, trunk, and limbs over the base of support. Then, the patient must learn to move in small increments in all directions over the base of support to relearn the postural adjustments that will eventually lead to balance reactions. When moving against gravity from sitting to standing, the patient will need much assistance. After work in standing, the patient should be able to take more control of postural alignment when returning to sitting, although some assistance may be necessary to maintain a better quality of movement and to keep the patient's weight centered over the base of support. It is important to remember that perfection of any of the above skills is achieved only by moving on to more advanced levels of skill or function. For example, taking the patient to standing and working on alignment in standing and control of weight-shifting will enable the patient to have more control in sitting, ie, the patient will have a more erect and symmetrical posture and be able to move more easily in all directions of sitting.

BASIC COMPONENTS OF MOVEMENT*

To develop postural stability with mobility, the ability to move in and out of postures (ie, transitional movements), and the ability to function in a posture, certain basic components of movement are necessary. These components enable us to control our bodies against gravity. Although listed and discussed separately, they are functionally inseparable.

Trunk Mobility and Control

As persons grow very old, they tend to lack stability and balance (related to disuse atrophy, disease, stress, etc.) and thus are less active and become less mobile; their muscles grow weaker. It is very important to help the older person to regain at least some mobility and strength to increase the ease of movement. Historically, in therapeutic exercise, the emphasized trunk movement has been rotation, but without the additional movements of anterior, posterior, and lateral pelvic tilts and free movement of the shoulder girdles, there is inadequate functional rotation. Recently, therefore, we have been placing more emphasis on the following movements to obtain more complete rotational ability: anterior and posterior tilt of the pelvis, upper back extension with shoulder girdle mobility, and the ability to shorten one side of the trunk and elongate the other by moving the pelvis on the thorax and laterally flexing the lumbar spine. Some elderly persons slump, making body movement in all directions very difficult. Most older persons tend to move the upper trunk and shoulders over the pelvis instead of moving the pelvis on the upper trunk, a movement necessary for normal balance reactions and general trunk adjustments when moving or using the limbs. This lack of trunk mobility makes limb function more difficult and disrupts head and neck alignment. Improvement of trunk mobility and control of the ensuing better alignment (ie, symmetry) improves all of the above. A better anterior tilt allows the person to develop better range and strength in upper back extension, which in turn helps head and neck alignment. (See *Head Control* section.) The anterior tilt and back extension enable the person to utilize the shoulder girdle more effectively, although it frequently is also necessary in the hemiplegic patient to inhibit spasticity in the shoulder girdle muscles. The ability to move and/or stabilize each shoulder girdle separately is particularly important for upper limb support and move-

---

* These components are well known, but grouping them in this manner was originally discussed by Cynthia S. Thomas and Jan Utley. The present discussion is an elaboration and expansion of those ideas by Jan Utley and myself.

ment. All the movements (anterior, posterior, and lateral tilt of the pelvis; shoulder girdle separation and stability) provide good functional rotation of the trunk and thus easier movement of head, trunk, and limbs in all directions.

The elderly stroke patient not only has trunk asymmetry and the lack of mobility and stability that frequently coincides with increasing age, but also has lost control of the limbs on one side of the body and, more important, the normal integration of the two sides of the trunk. This drastically affects the functioning of the whole body; regaining trunk and limb coordination that are as near normal as possible to make all movements easier becomes increasingly important. While trunk movements and symmetry are being improved, it is very important to help the patient reestablish motor control of the increased range and to be able to maintain a stable and more erect posture while moving the limbs selectively. The trunk movements must be incorporated into the normal daily activities. This increase in trunk mobility and stability in a more erect posture also improves respiratory function and generally enables all vital functions to be performed more effectively and efficiently. It is gratifying to hear patients comment on how good the additional movement in the trunk feels and to observe the change in affect within one or two sessions as movement becomes freer and more easily executed.

Head Control

As the elderly patient achieves control of a more mobile and better aligned trunk, the head is able to right more appropriately over the trunk. We discussed the trunk first because in older adults improving the trunk possture will almost always improve the head alignment but, as previously indicated, the control of both head and trunk are inseparable. If the head and neck are forward or tilted laterally, the posture of the trunk must be analyzed. A forward head often indicates a flexed trunk; a laterally tilted head frequently indicates a trunk that is laterally flexed. This is often just the normal righting of the head on a poorly aligned trunk. The trunk provides the base on which the head and limbs work; once the trunk is erect, the head tends to right itself. At times, if the neck has become stiff, one must gently assist the realignment while keeping the trunk erect and chin down. With the head and neck in better alignment over the trunk and a better balance of muscle tone in the trunk, the facial symmetry improves. The patient also swallows more effectively and has less chance of aspirating. One must not underestimate the importance of good head and trunk alignment, especially in the vertical posture.

Often, immobility in the shoulder girdle interferes with head and neck movements. This must be assessed because the head must be free to move independently (to turn, nod, etc.) without causing the trunk to move along with it. The head not only moves independently, but also influences movement in the rest of the body. For example, standing up becomes much easier if the head is lifted with some neck extension as one moves forward over the feet. Neck extension facilitates back extension, which in turn helps the legs be more dynamic and ready to push into extension to stand if the back extension is maintained as one bends at the hips.

Midline Orientation and Weight Shift

The key to controlling movement over the base of support is to establish the midline, ie, to recognize the middle and be able to center the body directly over one's base of support. Because we function primarily in vertical postures, midline orientation also means vertical orientation. All movement involves weight shift over the base of support. To develop balance, one must be able to align oneself symmetrically over one's base of support and shift in all directions with control. Stroke patients often have a disturbed sense of midline. Loss of sensation on the involved side, perceptual problems, and the asymmetry in hemiplegic patients resulting from an increase or decrease in postural tone in the trunk and limb muscles on the involved side contributes to this disturbed sense. Unless a good sense of midline is reestablished, balance is severely compromised, and the elderly patient may be unable to resume independent function safely. Because awareness of midline precedes the ability to be bilateral with one's limbs or to cross the midline, the lack of midline orientation results in inability to align the trunk symmetrically, to use both limbs together, or to cross one limb over the other while maintaining alignment, all of which interfere with function.

Limb Function

Two aspects of limb function must be considered: the ability to bear weight appropriately, and the ability to move the limb free in space. The weight-bearing component is developed first, and helps the infant acquire proximal stability both in the trunk and in the proximal joints of the limbs. Weight-bearing on the hand and foot helps the infant integrate the plantar and palmar reflexes and learn to control and grade movements of all joints in the limbs. Once that pattern becomes established, the infant has the ability to develop more skill and coordination of movements free in space. The developmental principle, "Weight-bearing precedes skilled coordinated movement," and the above mentioned aspects that are concomitant are just as applicable to elderly stroke patients and their recovery of function. Appropriate weight-bearing with good alignment and moving the body over the limb help to establish better tone, which in turn improves control in weight-bearing and movement. Using the limbs for the appropriate amount of support also provides better proximal stability with mobility and helps to inhibit the abnormal tone distally through open hand and total foot contact with the surface while establishing smooth controlled movement of the middle joint.

Once more normal tone has been achieved, the patient is assisted in the use of selective arm movements, often with the hand still in contact with a surface. For example, the patient learns to hold the arm at various points in the range of shoulder elevation while the hand is controlled by the therapist. This may be combined with a lengthening contraction (ie, lowering it into gravity in small increments). When these movements can be achieved with good quality, the patient is asked to raise it against gravity. All the movements must be performed without the patient going into abnormal movement patterns (ie, shoulder girdle retraction and elevation or depression or shoulder medial rotation, etc.); therefore, the therapists must grade their assistance very carefully and gradually withdraw it as the patient takes over more and more control. As control of one movement occurs, combining movements of one joint or two joints begins, progressing into the normal combination of movements in functional patterns. The patient may then begin utilizing the arm more naturally in daily function. Even a hand or arm with sensory deficits can become a supportive hand, although severe sensory loss definitely interferes with skilled use of the hand.

These components of movement have been listed separately only for clarity. In normal function, they are all utilized together regardless of the age of the adult. To achieve symmetry in the head and trunk, one must be able to achieve the midline. Normal weight shift requires midline orientation plus the ability to move well in all directions, which also requires head and trunk control. Using hand(s) and feet in weight-bearing can make development of head and trunk stability and mobility easier. Better head and trunk control and the ability to make postural adjustments augments skilled use of both arms and legs. The emphasis in treatment is on the whole body and the way in which all the parts contribute to a total activity or function. One must constantly assess and monitor the tone and movement patterns in the whole body and control abnormal tone and movement when necessary to achieve the best quality of function.

ASSESSMENT

The first assessment provides the basis with which later stages in the patient's condition can be compared. It also enables the therapist to determine primary problems and ways to begin changing them for the better. It is very important to establish early an effective means of communication with the patient. This can be verbal, manual, visual, or a combination of these, but it is essential that communication be established in order to evaluate and treat the patient adequately.

In the NDT (Bobath) approach, there is continual overlap between assessment and treatment throughout every treatment session. The therapist recognizes the responses of the patient and modifies the handling techniques accordingly to obtain continued improvement in the responses.

The following aspects of the approach need to be considered:

1. "Evaluation of postural tone and changes in tone which occur in different postures and situations.

2. Evaluation of the quality of the patient's postural and movement patterns.

3. Evaluation of his/her functional abilities and disabilities."[1]

A treatment plan can then be made, including the following general aims:

1. Increasing, decreasing, and/or stabilizing postural tone.

2. Determining which abnormal postural patterns or movement reactions should be inhibited and which normal patterns should be facilitated.

3. Deciding which functional skills the patient should be currently prepared for.[1]

TREATMENT

Most patients who have had a brain lesion, no matter what the cause, have abnormal tone and movement patterns. Following the assessment, the therapist should know the problems that exist and can begin treatment of the patient. As their approach evolved over the years, the Bobaths have kept normal postural tone against gravity as a baseline guide and have striven to achieve normal movement with their patients by a variety of handling techniques. Teaching patients to control and manage their own tone during daily functional activities is extremely important. The Bobaths say, "You cannot superimpose normal movement on abnormal tone." Thus, the primary element of the handling has been, to establish as near normal postural tone as possible. As a better balance of tone is achieved around the trunk, it becomes more symmetrical, and alignment over the hips can be maintained. This is essential for better functioning of the head and limbs as well as for controlling postures and moving between postures.

Once better postural tone is established, it is maintained while more normal movement patterns are facilitated. The therapist guides the patient in the function, facilitating the right components and controlling the tone when necessary to achieve success. This gives the patient the "feel" for more normal movement and helps to reestablish the appropriate sensation of the movement. When facilitating movement, one must wait for the patient to respond to one's handling. A lesioned brain requires longer to process information; therefore, the therapist must wait for the patient to respond in order to have the patient's active participation. Repetition, with gradually less control from the therapist, then usually makes it possible for the patient to reproduce the functional movement with components that are much more normal. With adults, the patterns most easily reestablished are basic functional activities such as transfers, trunk movements with and without arm support, coming to a standing or sitting position, gait, etc. Inhibition of abnormal tone and associated reactions* is accomplished by using weight-bearing on the limbs with good trunk and limb alignment as well as manual control at certain key points. Facilitating the essential components of the activity makes it easier for the patient and allows the therapist to provide enough assistance that the movements do not require excessive effort.

Initially, the therapist may control at more proximal key points (pelvis, shoulder girdle, etc.); as the patient gains more trunk stability and mobility, however, the therapist should move to more distal control points (arm, elbow, leg, knee, hand, or foot) to enable the patient to take over more whole body control. Proximal points of control do more to help the patient. Distal key points require more proximal control by the patient. No matter where the therapist's hands are used, control points must be varied and the therapist's control must be gradually removed as warranted; thus, the patient ultimately achieves independent function with movement patterns of good quality.

A key to achieving better functional movements is incorporating into all movement the essential components of balance and equilibrium reactions and protective extension of the arm. One utilizes balance reactions constantly. Those used most constantly are small trunk adjustments with weight shift around the midline and protective extension. Therefore, as the patient becomes ready, these responses are facilitated and built into the normal daily activities.

Berta Bobath also recognizes that the closer one gets to the actual functional situation while maintaining control of the abnormal tone, the better the carryover. To achieve this, there is continual overlap between assessment and treatment. She states:

> The therapist determines what makes the movement difficult or what is interfering with the patient's ability to carry out the desired movement. Then, she makes the movement possible by counteracting *anything* which interferes such as fear, lack of mobility, excessive tone or over-use of the good side. The therapist makes the movement possible by the way she handles the patient during the function. *The therapist is constantly in contact with the patient.* If the patient cannot understand what is said, communication still occurs through our hands guiding the patient through movement, through body language or through facial expressions. The therapist adapts the handling to the patient's response at the moment.

The therapist continually treats the responses of the patient as the patient functions, so that each treatment is individualized. If a therapist is walking a patient, the tone and associated reactions in the whole body must be monitored and controlled if necessary. For example, the arm should not be allowed to go into a flexion pattern. This associated reaction should be inhibited. Otherwise,

---

* Associated reactions are stereotyped postural patterns over which the patient has very little control. They are brought on by an effort or difficulty experienced by the patient. In hemiplegic patients, associated reactions produce a widespread increase in spasticity in the affected side.

the brain learns that the flexion pattern of the arm is a part of the gait pattern and it will thus be brain habituated. The more skillful the therapist is at making the appropriate adjustments (inhibitory and facilitatory) during the process of function, the better will be the quality of movement produced and the carryover achieved.

Grading and sequencing movements in functional activities is critical. All movements should be performed with limited effort by the patient, who must be actively involved; if the effort is too great, however, associated reactions and/or abnormal coordination of movement result. The therapist assists enough to control the abnormal responses and achieve good quality of movement. Then, as the patient begins taking over control of a posture and/or movement, the therapist *gradually* withdraws, thus helping the patient learn to grade and control the activity yet still maintain good quality movement. The subtle differences in the amount of pressure or assistance provided make the difference in the quality of the response. One can never be too skillful in this regard.

Often, the sequence of activities through which the patient is taken will determine the ultimate success or failure. For example, achieving some control of the trunk in sitting must be accomplished prior to scooting forward on a surface, one hip at a time. Some ability to bend forward at the hips with back extension is required to be able to slide the hips back on the surface pushing with both legs at the same time. These activities develop better tone in the trunk and legs, which will make transfers or coming to a standing position better and easier. Achieving and maintaining a more erect trunk posture and then relearning coordination between trunk and arm movements allow for easier and better quality arm patterns both in and out of weight bearing. As one continues to challenge patients at gradually higher levels, helping them achieve each activity with good quality, their lower level skills also improve. This point cannot be overemphasized. One's skill and abilities improve when one is challenged, but that challenge should be achievable and not so great that one is totally defeated.

Each step of the way, one tries to use the patients' abilities to help them accomplish more. A patient must achieve success in every session, as emotional state plays a key role in improvement of function. Excessive frustration or discouragement interferes with the ability to improve. It is not the patient's fault if the session is not successful; the fault lies in an unachievable goal within the time allotted or inadequate preparation of the patient. Being successful means accomplishing the activity with better components and with greater ease or achieving something not done previously, small though it may be.

Treatment should begin as soon as the patient is medically stable. The emphasis may initially be placed on positioning and bed mobility to assist patients in handling and moving their bodies in bed and on preventing contractures. This should be done slowly and with normal components so that the patient will be inclined to help automatically. As soon as possible, patients are brought to sitting and also to standing positions to reestablish the postures of function and to help restore vertical and midline orientation and general mental alertness. Using the upper and lower limbs for weight-bearing provides a natural support while helping patients regain trunk stability with mobility and preparing them for better overall limb function. If the therapist wants the patient to have good quality of movement for most activities of daily living (ADL), especially activities such as dressing, transfers, or coming to a standing position, a good base of support (ie, trunk mobility and stability) is necessary. This does not mean that ADL must be postponed until complete control is achieved, but it does mean that the appropriate trunk components and limb use must be facilitated during the process of each activity until patients can do it themselves with a better quality of movement.

Weight-bearing on the arm with the appropriate alignment in the limb helps develop shoulder girdle stability, which will decrease the possibility of shoulder subluxation. Until stability is achieved, the arm should be supported on a firm surface with the elbow slightly ahead of the shoulder and the shoulder joint in slight lateral rotation, if possible. Maintaining an erect trunk posture in both sitting and standing also facilitates better limb tone and better weight-bearing. To facilitate more dynamic back extension and thus a better sitting posture, a small lumbar pad may be used once lumbar extension is mechanically available. Sitting on a firm surface also improves posture.

All personnel working with patients should handle them in as similar a way as possible. These basics apply:

1.   Establish a need to look toward the involved side by placing interesting things on that side.

2.   In all daily care, patients should be given a chance and *time* to participate with some guidance in the movements. The key for therapists is usually doing it slowly so patients can help and in guiding them through the movements.

3.   Remember that expecting cognitive as well as motor improvement simultaneously in dressing, for instance, may be too overwhelming and frustrating to patients. Reestablish the movement patterns for dressing before requiring right, left, front, and back concepts.

Throughout all aspects of treatment, one must constantly be striving to improve balance. This is the biggest problem for all stroke patients and for most elderly people as well because of their decrease in activity and general mobility. (Note: According to C. C. Conrad, Executive Director of the United States President's Council of Physical Fitness and Sports, the balance mechanism is maintained through use and degenerates when not used. Many older people are more vulnerable to losing their sense of balance, especially those who use eye glasses and hearing aids.)[2] Improving trunk mobility and stability improves sitting balance. When patients are ready, standing and walking balance must be specifically addressed to help decrease their fear. Patients with adult hemiplegia have a very great fear of falling; in addition, they fear that once they are down, they will not be able to get up. Therefore, teaching the patients how to get up from the floor will relieve some of their fear. One cannot eliminate fear; everyone experiences it. But one can certainly decrease fear, thereby lessening the severity of increased tone and abnormal movement patterns that occur in stroke patients.

The speed and degree of recovery of function depends largely on the severity of the lesion and the type of input the patient receives. We do know there is much more potential in the brain for recovery of function than was previously believed. Many factors (age, nutrition, location of the lesion, cohort support, etc.)[3] ultimately determine the patient's recovery. Our job as therapists is to identify those factors interfering with normal motor function and to attempt to diminish or eliminate them while helping patients reestablish the previously learned functional patterns.

Some stroke patients have flaccidity or true muscle weakness. Often, this weakness is from disuse and/or a loss of the memory of movement patterns. The brain does not remember how to move. Reestablishing the sensory-motor input by passively moving the affected part of the body often enables the patient to assist with the movement. Sometimes, putting the limb in a weight-bearing position in which it would normally be used activates the anti-gravity muscles, and the patient begins to support with the limb. Strengthening in this treatment approach is done through normal functional activities using the appropriate muscle groups to perform the components of the activity. Exercise and weight programs used to strengthen the better limbs encourage associated reactions and abnormal tone on the involved side. Strengthening programs for the involved side accentuate abnormal patterns and may eliminate the potential for selective movement on that side. Therefore, *we discourage resistive exercise programs as much as possible.*

ADDITIONAL PROBLEMS

Pain

Patients often have pain, which interferes with recovery of function. The most common cause of pain in the hemiplegic shoulder is increased tone in the shoulder girdle muscles. This can often be relieved by inhibiting the excessive tone unless there has been some trauma or damage to the tissues around the shoulder. Inhibition of the shoulder girdle muscles by slow, small easy movements of the scapula tends to decrease pain, and thus may be the initial preferable treatment. Caution should be exercised, and staying *below* the pain threshold must be emphasized. Pain may also be present in the upper arm, forearm, or hand when the arm hangs dependent for long periods of time. Supporting the arm on a table or lap board should help to relieve this if the surface is the appropriate height. Premorbid conditions such as arthritis or bursitis in or around various joints will also contribute to the pain syndrome. No matter where the pain is, it must be relieved before therapy can progress.

Overactivity of the Sound Side

Patients overuse their better side because they feel unstable in the trunk or lack balance. One must diminish the overuse, but better stability in the trunk must first be achieved. As patients gain in trunk control, they tend to use the sound limbs less and rely more on their trunk muscles for balance. It is extremely important to accomplish trunk control because any overuse of the good limbs results in associated reactions or abnormal responses in the involved limbs. Reestablishing a better balance of tone in both limbs and gaining bilateral support early will help patients use both sets of limbs more effectively and appropriately.

Loss of Sensation

Patients have varying degrees of sensory loss which influences the way they respond. The therapist must keep two important factors in mind when considering sensation. First, with appropriate weight-bearing on the limb, patients may achieve better awareness, which will improve automatic responses. Second, sensory testing assesses primarily cortical awareness of sensation, not sensation that is received, processed, and responded to at a subcortical level. It is important to test both movement and position sense initially to determine the degree of proprioceptive input. Initially tactile sensation must also be tested, particularly light and deep pressure. Testing temperature, two-point discriminations and stereognosis may be more appropriate when the patient is ready to begin using the hand for skilled movements. Sensory loss will interfere with high level hand function, but it is possible for a patient to develop a useful supportive hand in spite of a fairly severe sensory loss. It is important to achieve good alignment and appropriate weight-bearing on the limb to achieve maximum results.

Multiple Diagnoses

Elderly stroke patients often have premorbid medical conditions or other diagnoses, in addition to the stroke. Each patient must be assessed individually, taking all physical, cognitive, and emotional conditions into consideration. The handling (therapeutic intervention) will be determined by the therapist based on how the patient responds to what is done. There is no set exercise routine that can apply to all or even most patients. All individuals are different; thus, all handling will be different. No matter what the problem(s), the therapist should strive for the best possible tone and the highest possible level of function of which the individual is capable.

Documentation

Recording progress is a task every therapist faces, and the key to effective documentation is for therapists to select goals so precisely that they know the goals can be accomplished in the desired time frame. Writing each goal specifically as accurate and meaningful documentation reflects the real skill of the therapist.

In summary, the NDT (Bobath) approach is applicable to the elderly stroke patient. The approach keeps the patient's effort level to a minimum while the patient works on basic functional skills necessary for daily living. The therapy session may be built around the accomplishment of a specific function, such as a transfer with good quality of movement. For example, the ability to scoot forward and back on a surface is worked on, as is each of the movement components as necessary. Then, the transfer is done in small increments, incorporating weight-bearing on both upper and lower limbs. (Note: This transfer is done as a normal person would move from one surface to another, not as a standing pivot transfer.) This enables the patient to gain better control of the whole body while also relearning to transfer easily. The problems interfering with the patient's ability to perform the function are identified; the patient is then guided through the movement while the abnormal tone and movement patterns are inhibited whenever and wherever necessary. The highest level of function possible is emphasized to improve the patients' control and to help them progress as rapidly as possible. The ultimate goal is safe, independent function with good quality of movement patterns.

REFERENCES

1. Bobath B: Adult Hemiplegia: Evaluation and Treatment. 2nd Ed. Heinemann Medical Books, London, 1978
2. Conrad C. C: Regular exercise program is beneficial psychologically as well as physically. Geriatrics 29:40, 1974
3. Finger S, Stein D: Brain Damage and Recovery: Research and Clinical Implications. Academic Press, Orlando, FL, 1982

12 | Progressive Exercise Program: A Model Approach for Working with Elderly Patients

Georgiana W. Johnson

UNDERSTANDING POSTURE AND GAIT TRAINING

In assuming a position vertical to space and gravity, a person starts to develop individuality in posture and gait. The upright posture is a learned behavior influenced by genetic factors, attitudes, and parental models, as well as by the overall neuromusculoskeletal system as it relates to gravity. Deviations from the accepted norm may be caused by a variety of factors, such as injury, poor habits, inadequate nutrition, depression, or a distorted image of what is "correct." (This distorted image leads to a constant attempt to stand and walk in a certain way, such as the exaggerated military stance or placing one foot in front of the other, as models are often taught.)

Whether a certain posture and gait evolve from one's conscious or unconscious actions, the results are the same; deep-rooted *habits that "feel right to the individual."* These habits often contribute to misuse, abuse, and injury, resulting in a variety of symptoms, such as fatigue, ineffective movement, reduced productivity, and pain. These symptoms may be connected to common emotional overlays of depression, anxiety, dissatisfaction, skepticism, disenchantment, and with a failure to find acceptable cures or answers to the problems.

Mild posture and gait dysfunctions are often the early warning signs with which a physical therapist is asked to work. Effective treatment of posture and gait dysfunctions in the elderly patient takes more time in each session than is commonly alloted in many physical therapy settings. Assessing the early symptoms of posture and gait dysfunctions requires that the therapist have great skill because the clinical manifestations are not predictable and are often unique to each individual patient (especially in the elderly). The therapist may initially obtain an unsatisfactory result from traditional physical therapy modalities (ie, heat, strength exercises, etc.).

We must ask ourselves what is wrong. Is it our evaluation, program planning, support system, expectations, lack of interest, or lack of time? To justify our frustations we can think of many possible reasons, including: "The patient did not follow directions." But, indirectly, therapists must also assume the responsibility for any treatment program that does not achieve the desired therapeutic outcome. A poor therapeutic outcome may be fostered by the choice of ineffective exercises, inappropriate methods of presentation, use of ineffective communication with the patient, or by a motivational approach that does not meet the individual needs of the patient. Evaluation cannot be overemphasized; however, implementation of an effective therapeutic program is the essential component of treatment. Many good books focus on what exercises "to do," but the "how to do" and the "motivation to do" have not been given enough attention; this is especially important when working with older patients. Perhaps this deficit evolves from the assumption that patients will automatically apply useful analytical knowledge in their daily lives. This assumption is as unrealistic as expecting a person to read a book or to buy the best golf clubs and win the U.S. Open golf championship the following week.

A program does not become effective for a patient until it has minimized or displaced poor and ineffective habits and replaced them with more mechanically and neurologically sound habits. It is not advisable to change a person's habit without developing a better replacement.[1] The patient's old habits of alignment "*feel right*" and are perpetuated by the *automatic computer brain* and the way it has been *programmed*. If we hope to change old habits, we must identify undesirable movement habits and reprogram the brain so that the new posture and desired movements will not only feel better, but feel right. The Progressive Exercise Program (PEP) focuses on *how*—the actual details of the way to carry out the therapeutic process.

UNDERSTANDING THERAPEUTIC CONCEPTS

Many kinds of exercises exist, and most of them are good for something or someone. Not all exercises are good for everything and everyone, however. Exercises can be structured to achieve a variety and/or a combination of goals, including increase of:

1. Strength
2. Mobility
3. Range of motion
4. Flexibility
5. Stability
6. Agility
7. Aerobic reactions
8. Relaxation and release of tension

The ultimate goal of therapeutic intervention is to reduce symptoms, improve function, and develop a maintenance program to prevent future problems and/or regression to ineffective movement patterns. Physical therapists provide exercise programs based on the physician's diagnosis and request for therapeutic intervention. Physical therapists have been trained in rehabilitation exercise techniques in their formal education and through on-the-job experience and continuing education courses. Some therapists have studied other treatment approaches, such as yoga, Tai-Chi, Aston Patterning, Feldenkrais Method, and others, that have developed outside the medical profession.

PEP evolved from a firm neurological background and has been enhanced by careful implementation of chosen concepts and techniques from traditional and nontraditional sources into a unique program designed to be adapted to each individual patient's needs. PEP was designed primarily to improve postural alignment and to develop better dynamics of gait and body mechanics. It is not an end but rather a beginning for forming the foundation from which other types of physical activities can evolve and expand. Optimally, these functional activities will develop in harmony with gravity and within each individual's personal limitations, capacities, and needs. Once a person has a good basis for movement in harmony with gravity, all motor skills will improve, require less effort, and be more enjoyable. For these reasons, PEP is presented as a model program of therapeutic intervention for the elderly. However, PEP is a relevant therapeutic program adaptable for any age group.

Implications For Therapy

In structuring a therapeutic exercise program, one should consider the following questions as they relate to each individual patient:

1. What are the patient's motivational factors?
2. What are the patient's needs? Has the evaluation of posture and gait identified the alignment, function, and abilities of the entire body?
3. Are the choices of exercises individualized and compatible with the patient's habits and needs?
4. Are the therapeutic expectations realistic?
5. Is the manner of executing the exercises structured to make them effective and easy to perform?

6. Can the patient understand and feel comfortable with the new concepts?

UNDERSTANDING THE AGING PROCESS

Four significant factors that we cannot change influence posture and gait function. The first is the earth's gravitational force, and the second is the aging process. These two factors combine to decrease functional capacity and increase vulnerability to fatigue, injuries, and decreased productivity. The other factors over which we have no control are individual genetic makeup and body build, and parental models. Posture and gait are characteristic of each individual and function on an automatic level that has evolved from repetition over time. These patterns may be mechanically sound and contribute to a desirable appearance and function. If the habitual patterns are imbalanced, some muscles become weak and others become tight or shortened, contributing to poor function and appearance and accelerating the functional losses with the aging process. Obesity and weight-related problems accompanying aging often create joint stress and intensify posture and gait dysfunction. To cope with these

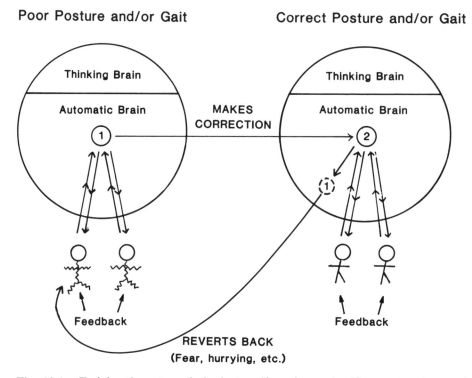

Fig. 12-1. Training the automatic brain to self-monitor and self-correct posture and gait.

problems, the neuromusculoskeletal system must be trained or retrained to self-monitor and self-correct posture and gait (Fig. 12-1).

1. Old habit *computer chip* that feels right.
2. New habit *computer chip* that has been learned to replace the old undesirable chip.

The old habit computer chip will over-ride the new one as a function of fatigue, hurrying, anger, etc. The brain, however, has the capacity to perceive this by self-monitoring and self-correcting, forming the basis for new habits and improving function and the ability to decelerate the aging process by controlling the neuromusculoskeletal system and minimizing the negative effects of gravity.

UNDERSTANDING INTERNAL AWARENESS FOR POSTURAL ALIGNMENT

Traditionally, postural alignment is judged by external appearance of the body, and corrections are focused on external adjustments. "Put your shoulders back;" "Do a pelvic tilt," and "Straighten up," are typical verbal suggestions we give ourselves and others. We also look in a mirror or a store window to see if we are standing "straight." Unfortunately, these methods are not as effective as we would like. They usually foster overcorrection and persist only as long as we are consciously thinking about maintaining the change.

We must utilize our subconscious as a means to self-monitor and self-correct to maintain continual optimal adjustments and control of postural function through the neuromusculoskeletal systems. Thus, therapeutic intervention must create a subconscious (internal) reference point for the desired alignment. The brain must develop the ability to monitor incoming sensory information from the body and accept or reject it. If the information is rejected, the brain must make the necessary corrections to match the preestablished reference point. Each of us has the capacity to develop *body feedback* to achieve this need. We must train the automatic system and program our brain to self-monitor and to self-correct.

Implications for Therapy

1. Accept the importance of internal awareness of movements and create the desire to acquire the skill of self-monitoring and self-correcting.
2. Accept the responsibility of devoting the necessary time to train and maintain the monitoring system, and practice the PEP designed to meet individual needs at least 1 hour daily for the first 3 months and then for 30 minutes to 1 hour three or four times a week as a maintenance program (as needed).

3. Develop rhythm, repetition, and reciprocation in exercises and feel the carryover into all activities of daily living (ADL).

4. Be aware of factors that cause regression to old habits, such as fatigue, hurrying, anger, tension, pain, certain positions, and certain people.

5. Because it takes time to replace old habits and practice to establish and maintain new postural and movement habits one must stay mentally, physically, and emotionally tuned-in to creating an awareness and a reference point on the automatic level.

6. Recognize when the body slips back into old undesirable habits and immediately make the necessary corrections (self-monitor, self-correct).

UNDERSTANDING TEACHING AND LEARNING PRINCIPLES

The basic concept of the famous educator John Dewey is that we learn to do by doing. It has been said that, we understand what we hear, believe what we see, but do not learn until we *do*. A habit is not established until it is performed repetitively in a comfortable way, thus programming it to be performed on the automatic level. The law of readiness states that learning happens more easily when a person is motivated to make a change. An effective therapist is a guide and an instructor who educates and motivates a patient to change, thus decreasing dependency and increasing independence.

Implications for Therapy

1. Create a quiet, calm, comfortable environment for working with the patient.

2. Use relaxing background music and/or tape-recorded instructions for home programs.

3. Use imagery to enhance the mental picture of positions and movements.

4. Use a nurturing touch. Adapt touch to each patient's tolerance and acceptance. Use touch to locate and guide movement, direction, amplitude, and resistance when indicated.

5. Stress key words and present helpful suggestions, such as: "Easy knees," "Release," "Allow the body to," "Feel heavy," "Feel light," etc.

6. Use successive approximation—approach each goal slowly, a little at a time.

7. Work with an amount of time as opposed to a specific number of repetitions. Each exercise should incorporate the entire body, identifying clearly the body parts functioning as a stabilizer and those functioning as prime movers.

8. Utilize frequent rest periods. One learns faster with intermittent rest periods. During rest, one may use imagery of the desired movement, which can act as an adjunct to facilitating the ease of mastering the real movement.

9.   Reinforce results with a good feeling of accomplishment and ask the patient to monitor and compare, developing the ability to perceive the differences that are created as being increasingly balanced in relation to gravity. Create an awareness of feeling lighter and of perceiving an automatic flow of walking with rhythm, which occurs without conscious effort.

10.   Structure all exercises from a neuromusculoskeletal orientation, developing automatic internal–external awareness for the desired alignment and movements.

UNDERSTANDING PEP

PEP evolved as an effective way to develop integrated movement of the body in harmony with gravity. It is not meant to be the *end* of exercises, but rather the *foundation* from which other appropriate exercises and activities can evolve and expand.

PEP can function as a corrective, a therapeutic, and/or a maintenance program, depending on the needs of each individual as determined by the complete posture and gait evaluation by a physical therapist. PEP can be structured and taught individually or in groups, helping each individual to adapt to specific needs.

All PEP exercises are structured to have four degrees of difficulty. Programs are designed, individualized, and progressed to meet each patient's needs. Cassette tapes are issued to be used daily as home programs. Patients are taught body mechanic techniques that utilize new improved functional capacities in ADL, work, and recreational activities.

Once coordinated movement (a balance of muscular length, strength, and timing of activation) is possible, all activities become easier and more enjoyable. An awareness of feeling in better alignment and functioning without conscious effort serves as a motivating factor for patients to continue the daily maintenance program. Figure 12-2 gives examples of basic PEP exercise positions which form the foundation from which other exercises evolve and progress to develop an internal awareness of optimal alignment and coordination of patterns of motion, including the reciprocal walking pattern. When a patient adheres to a 60-minute daily period of structured PEP exercises that incorporate the entire body, the patient automatically starts standing and walking in better alignment and often asks: "How can so little do so much, when so much I have done has done so little?" The therapist can answer: "You have trained and programmed the total neuromusculoskeletal system to operate on the automatic level and to self-monitor and self-correct."

UNDERSTANDING BASIC PRINCIPLES
Basic Learning Principles for PEP

1.   The PEP exercise program must be experienced in order to understand its effectiveness. Do not attempt to teach it until you have performed it often enough to appreciate its biological and mechanical significance.

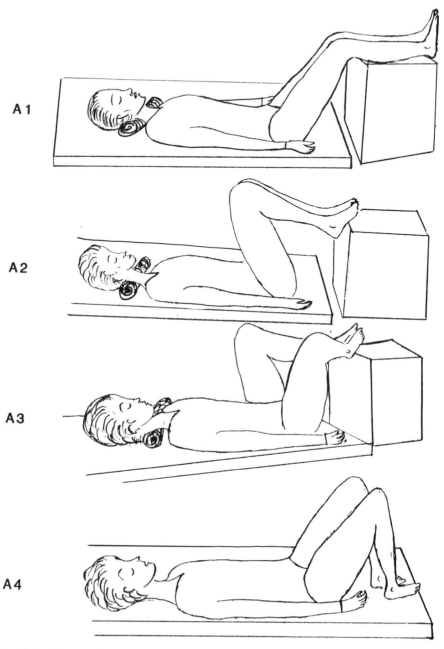

Fig. 12-2. Progressive exercise program. (PEP). Progression I: A1, A2, A3, A4. These positions enhance optimal postural alignment and form a baseline for progression of PEP exercises to evolve from supine, to sitting, standing, and walking.

2. Time is an important factor—the movements should be executed slowly, allowing time between repetitions for release of tension throughout the body. An exercise period should be a minimum of 30 to 60 minutes to allow time for the body to adapt and establish internal awareness. Time is needed to change old alignment and movement habits and replace them with more comfortable and desirable habits. Once a maintenance level has been established, time should be set aside for daily periods of exercise.

3. Progression should be structured to start at a low degree of difficulty and advance slowly. Criteria for moving to the next progression include control of stability and ease of movement for 1 week prior to advancing, and ability to use movements within a pain-free range.

4. Observe the laws of readiness and motivation—the patient should feel emotionally and psychologically prepared to participate (see Chapter 1, Staging for Bond of Trust).

5. Practice and repetition are necessary to change old habits into new ones and maintain them. Motion must be controlled and practiced in a correct manner to develop internal awareness. Exercises that are executed mechanically or that fail to focus on internal awareness and feedback will be less effective.

6. An act becomes automatic as a function of repetition in a controlled comfortable manner accompanied by pleasant and accepting attitudes.

7. Skill is more likely to be retained if daily exercise periods are observed.

Basic Biological Principles for PEP

1. Motor output is affected by sensory input.

2. The body has an internal feedback system for self-monitoring and self-correcting.

3. Proprioceptors are located in the muscles, tendons, and joints. They control posture and movement.

4. Many proprioceptors function on an automatic (subconscious) level.

5. Respiration and circulation work together to supply the body tissues with required oxygen and nutrients to carry away waste materials.

6. Muscles act in patterns of motions. These patterns can be superimposed on the system to help form new habits and replace old habits.

Basic Mechanical Principles for PEP

1. The gravitational force of the earth interacts with the muscular actions of the body to determine position and time in space and their derivatives (x, displacement; $\dot{x}$, velocity; and $\ddot{x}$, acceleration).

2. The greatest efficiency of movement and stability is achieved when the body alignment is in harmony with gravity.

3. The position of the center of gravity changes with every change of body position.

4. The state of equilibrium of the human body depends on the height of the center of gravity, the location of the line of gravity in relation to the base of the support, the size of the supporting base and the external forces acting on the body.

5. A large base of support is more stable than a small base.

6. The body is more stable when the center of gravity is directly over the supporting base.

7. A triangular or a three-point support is more stable than a straight line (a two-point support).

8. Greater efficiency of movement is achieved when all musculoskeletal forces are in the direction of the intended motion.[2]

Implications for Therapy

1. The body must develop a reference point of internal awareness for the alignment of each segment in relation to the segments above and below.

2. When the body is in an upright position, the center of gravity in the frontal plane should be lowered; for example, slightly drop the buttocks toward the heels and the knees toward the toes.

3. Therapy must work with alignment of the entire body, not just one segment, such as the low back or the painful area.

4. When walking, focus the force for momentum and control to come from the push-off of the forefoot and toes.

UNDERSTANDING HABITS: A BASIC PREMISE IN PEP

A habit, with regard to posture and gait, is unique to each individual. Habits adapt and change as functions of time and circumstances. Sometimes we are aware of a habit and recognize it as desirable or undesirable. If it is undesirable we may want to change it or choose to accept it as being normal for us. We often expect other people to accept us as we are, and we rationalize that the old habitual alignment is what feels right. *Corrected* posture that has been superimposed externally by means of will power before an internal awareness is achieved is not only perceived by the individual as "feeling weird" but is rejected as undesirable.

Postural and gait habits perpetuate on an automatic (subconscious) level. They do not become firmly established overnight and cannot be changed overnight. Postural habits may deviate from the accepted normal limits without causing pain or problems. Persons with such habits may be satisfied with their bodies and not feel the need or the desire to change. They may be more vulnerable to fatigue and accidents, as a result of poor body mechanics and mechanical stress related to the minor postural deviations.

When postural alignment and poor body mechanics contribute to pain, a vicious cycle begins, perpetuating and intensifying pain. *Malalignment causes pain and pain causes malalignment.* This type of problem usually motivates a person to seek help and to make changes to alleviate pain and improve quality of life. But how can habits be changed?

The individual involved must:

1. Accept the need and the desire to change.
2. Recognize that he or she does not know how to change and then seek help from a reliable source.
3. Be aware that many exercise programs are not appropriate and may even cause more problems.

Guideliness for an appropriate program include the following suggestions:

1. Establish an internal reference point for correct posture and gait.
2. Adapt correction to each person's capacity to self-monitor and self-correct.
3. Choose exercises that will place the body in desired positions to develop a comfortable feeling that acts as a reference point for stabilization and controlled movement.
4. Present the exercise program in a manner that facilitates reorganization of the neuromuscular patterns of stability and movement and facilitates a sense of ease *physically and emotionally*.

In summary, success in changing habits depend on:

1. A true desire combined with sustained motivation.
2. A program that is individually designed and implemented to replace undesirable habits with desirable new ones.
3. The accuracy and consistency with which the program is executed.
4. The use of rhythm, repetition, and reciprocation in formulating new habits.
5. The development of awareness and ability to self-monitor and self-correct.

Remember: It takes time and repetition of new habits to replace old ones.

UNDERSTANDING BREATHING CONCEPTS IN PEP

Breathing is necessary for sustaining life. How we breathe influences our quality of life. Breathing reflects our innermost feelings. It is a function of our autonomic system; however, we are able to exert conscious control to influence its rate and depth and the area of chest expansion and diaphragm action.

Much emphasis has been placed on inhalation and getting air into the lungs.

Many times, inhalation is repeated without adequate exhalation to remove all of the "old air" from the lungs and make room for fresh air. Learning to place emphasis on controlled exhalation and abdominal-diaphragmatic control facilitates release of physical and mental tension and promotes relaxation.

Implications for Therapy

1.   Diaphragmatic-abdominal breathing should be developed with emphasis on exhalation and allowing inhalation to happen automatically (presuming that there is adequate expansion of rib cage and absence of using accessory breathing muscles.) In most older clients this is not the case, and basic intervention is required to decrease involvement of accessory breathing muscles (see Chapter 4).

2.   When a person exercises, breathing can combine inhalation with initiation of movement, and exhalation with release of movement or be purposefully allowed to function undisturbed by the exercise. (This sequence is reversed for some abdominal exercises.) Breathing should always be executed with rhythm and with ease.

3.   Slow breathing can be used to enhance the ability to relax and to release tension and induce sleep.

UNDERSTANDING EVALUATION

All therapeutic exercise plans are based on clinical evaluation and knowledge of normal and abnormal function of the body. Extensive research and years of clinically derived knowledge from analysis of normal and abnormal posture and gait problems are well documented in the literature.

Perry,[3] Inman,[4] Kendall,[5] Hellebrandt,[6] and others have made valuable contributions through publications, teaching, and by clinically sharing information and training others to carry on their work. They all focus on evaluating, identifying problems, and providing corrective programs for improved function.

Evaluation of posture and gait can be compared with solving a jig-saw puzzle. All parts are present but they may not be arranged optimally. A single piece of the puzzle is dependent on the alignment of three or four pieces, which are in turn dependent on three or four more adjacent pieces. The puzzle cannot be completed until every piece is adapted to be compatible with the total puzzle. Application of this concept to the evaluation and treatment of body posture and body mechanics means that we must look beyond the painful area. To emphasize the importance of total body control, the therapist might ask the patient: "When building a house, would you try to put the roof on before laying the foundation?" The therapist might add, "If you had a sore toe it would hurt, but if someone stepped on it, it would hurt more."

Is there a missing piece to the puzzle in the evaluation process? What does the therapist use to enhance the patient outcome?

1. We depend on vision to identify external images.

2. We depend on auditory perceptors in judging deviations in how the body contacts the floor; (ie, Do the heels strike the floor too hard? Does the forefoot slap the floor? Is there symmetry in the step length and duration?)

3. We depend on our tactile receptors in making judgments by palpation and muscle testing. All these perceptions are external observations of internal functions.

4. Through x-ray films, electromyogram (EMG) studies, computed axial tomography (CAT) scans, and thermograms, we obtain information regarding internal conditions and deficits.

Therefore, what piece of the puzzle is missing? The missing piece of information is *patients' awareness of their postural alignment and function*, the state of internal kinesthetic awareness. Assessment of the patients' kinesthetic awareness can be included with other subjective judgments, including attitudes, depression, self-image, and the motivation to make the evaluation process complete. A patient who is dealing with marked pathological deviations does not find it difficult to feel what is happening and to recognize and accept the need for change. The patient is also able to perceive feeling differently in a positive way as changes occur. It is difficult for the therapist to perceive the patient's deviate patterns internally and reproduce them externally. Therapists sometimes expect patients to make changes from visual and auditory cues before they have facilitated the appropriate internal kinesthetic awareness and therefore are disappointed with the patients' failure to make the desired changes.

For every person with pathological gait and postural deviations, there are hundreds of people with mechanical postural and gait deviations. Many such persons continue to function forever at a level at which they can adapt and cope. Others, through continued misuse, abuse, and/or injury, develop symptoms that bring them to the medical profession for help. When this type of patient is evaluated, the therapist benefits by being able to reproduce the detail of the postural and gait patterns. The ability to mimic the details of a movement pattern allows the therapist to determine how it feels and what movement and alignment changes make a difference. This input helps form the basis for program planning. When a therapist attempts to reproduce an observed gait and posture, the deviations will most likely be exaggerated and not photographically identical. With practice, the therapist can gradually approximate the deviations. Some therapists, however, may reply, ''I can't walk that way; my body does not cooperate.'' We often expect our patients to implement changes before we have helped them acquire an internal awareness for self-monitoring and self-correcting.

''I've shown you what to do, I told you what to do, and I have given you a book to read—now do it.'' This approach sets our patients up for failure and sends them out to shop for another physician, another therapist, and a perpetuation of their problem. *The internal sensory integrity of our patients must be included in our evaluation and treatment plan.* The therapist must learn to internalize and reproduce the deviate postural and gait patterns to enhance the understanding of the total problem in order to design and implement effective programs. Until we incorporate these elements into our evaluation and treatment plans, we will continue to work in a hit-or-miss fashion, at least much of the time.

CONCLUSION

The PEP exercise program offers a therapeutic regimen that is built on conscious expansion of a patient's internal sensory awareness and posture/movement.

PEP helps the participant progress through an appropriate exercise regimen as the patient's kinesthetic awareness matures. PEP offers specific literature designed for both the therapist's needs and the patient's needs.[7]

REFERENCES

1. Goffman E: Asylums. Anchor Books, Garden City, NY, 1961
2. Smith, H: Introduction to Human Movement. p. 31. Addison-Wesley, Reading, MA, 1968
3. Perry J, Antonelli D, Ford W: Analysis of knee-joint forces during flexed-knee stance, *J Bone Joint Sur* 57–A:961, 1975
4. Inman VT, Ralston NJ, Todd F: Human Walking. Williams & Wilkins, Baltimore, 1981
5. Kendall HO, Florence P, Wadsworth GE: Muscles, Testing, and Function. Williams & Wilkins, Baltimore, 1971
6. Hellebrandt FA, Houtz SJ, Eubank: Influence of alternate and reciprocal exercises on work capacity. Arch Phys Med, 32:766, 1951
7. Johnson G. W: PEP (manuscript in preparation)

Index

Page numbers followed by *f* indicate figures; those followed by *t* indicate tables.